First published in 2006 by
Darton, Longman and Todd Ltd
1 Spencer Court
140–142 Wandsworth High Street
London SW18 4JJ

Reprinted 2006 (twice)

ISBN–10: 0–232–52687–7
ISBN–13: 978–0–232–52687–5

talogue record for this book is available from the British Library.

Designed by Sandie Boccacci
Typeset by YHT Ltd, London
Printed and bound in Great Britain by
The Cromwell Press, Trowbridge, Wiltshire

The Enduring Melody

The Enduring M

MICHAEL MAYNE

Also by Michael Mayne:

A Year Lost and Found
This Sunrise of Wonder
Pray, Love, Remember
Learning to Dance

DARTON · LONGMAN + TO

In memory of four valued friends

Stewart
John
Giles
Terence

who died too young,
claimed – though not defeated – by cancer

Think where man's glory most begins and ends,
And say my glory was I had such friends.
W. B. Yeats[1]

CONTENTS

God guard me from those thoughts men think
In the mind alone;
He that sings a lasting song
Thinks in the marrow-bone.

W. B. Yeats[2]

I ponder all the possibilities that come with being human. Good and evil, happiness and misery, achievement and failure, love and isolation – everything that goes into being the particular person you are in that particular social and historical setting. That's a lot, isn't it? My God, that's some menu!

William Boyd[3]

What a little vessel of strangeness we are, sailing through this muffled silence through the autumn dark.

Max in John Banville's The Sea

All Mankind is of one Author, and is in one volume; when one Man dies, one Chapter is not torn out of the book, but translated into a better language; and every Chapter must be so translated; God employs several translators; some pieces are translated by age, some by sickness, some by war, some by justice; but God's hand is in every translation; and his hand shall bind up all our scattered leaves again, for that library where every book shall lie open to one another.

John Donne[4]

FOREWORD

The Enduring Melody is an inspired choice of title for an inspiring book, which can help readers of all religions and none to get in touch with the enduring melody of their own lives, a melody which permeates every moment, both of darkness and light. Moments of our own lives which, at the time, were dissonant and threatening, become woven by the enduring melody into a wider, more expansive, more universal context, setting us free to glimpse and delight in the mystery in which all of us live and move and have our being.

'The enduring melody' is a translation of the Latin term *cantus firmus*, which we call 'plain chant' – a fixed song, the music of the monasteries. This later developed into polyphony: many different voices singing in harmony and counterpoint around the main melody. Events in our lives and the words which describe the events can be compared to musical notes which weave in and out of the enduring melody.

The Enduring Melody is rich in apt quotations which never distract from, but always confirm the main theme. One of the most apt is from William Byrd, the sixteenth-century English composer, who wrote:

> There is a certain hidden power in the thoughts underlying the words themselves, so that as one meditates and constantly and seriously considers them, the right notes in some inexplicable fashion suggest themselves spontaneously.

There is a mysterious connection between actions, words and music, so we speak of a 'sound person', of a person who 'rings true', of 'harmony between nations'. In reading any book or article, it is good to ask oneself, 'How does it sound to you?' The question is especially useful after reading *The Enduring Melody*. For me, it has been like listening to a symphony in printed words. It rings true, full of counterpoint as Michael faces 'the country of cancer in his own life', experiences the stripping away of all that supports him in life, the physical pain, the experience of utter helplessness and terrifying fear as he suffers drug-induced hallucinations and feels he is losing his mind. In his agony and torment he keeps in touch with that enduring melody, faint and fragile in his consciousness at times, but which allows him to thank God for the cancer, not in itself, but in its effect on him, bringing him more in touch with the enduring melody that is the intimate presence of God with him always, accompanying him in his sense of abandonment.

The Enduring Melody does not only explore the country of cancer: through his own life experience, Michael has many reflections on God, Jesus, prayer, the Church; on art, poetry and love. One could easily forgive an elderly man who had suffered so much for rambling in vague reflections on such central topics, but Michael's reflections are full of wisdom and insight into the wonderful mystery of our lives. The high points of his symphony are often contained in his reflections. God is in all things and God's incarnation is not limited to the Word made flesh in Jesus, for as Gerard Manley Hopkins wrote: 'Christ plays in ten thousand places, lovely in limbs, lovely in eyes not his'.

In his postscript to the book, Michael writes:

> However mixed our motives in writing (or reading) books, in the end they are about our desire to share (and learn more about) what it means to be human and what matters to us most, our desire 'to speak what we feel, not what we ought to say'. For those who write such books, and nervously launch them into a critical world, they aim to be, in short, a small – and sometimes quite risky – act of love.

Thank you, Michael, for your risk of love, for what better gift could you leave us than this testament, which can help us to become more aware of our own enduring melody, a melody that points us, as it has pointed you, beyond ourselves to glimpse the all-embracing, self-giving mystery in which we all live, move and have our being, the desire of all our desiring.

Gerard W. Hughes SJ
June 2006

ACKNOWLEDGEMENTS

The publisher is grateful for permission to reprint extracts from the following:

W. H. Auden, 'Lullaby', from *Thank You, Fog*, Faber and Faber, 1974. Used by permission of Faber and Faber Ltd.

John Burnside, 'Kith', from *The Light Trap*, published by Jonathan Cape, reprinted by permission of the Random House Group Ltd.

Raymond Carver, 'Late Fragment', from *All of Us*, published by Harvill, reprinted by permission of The Random House Group Ltd.

Padraig Daly, 'Trinity', from *The Other Sea*, Dedalus Press, 2003. Used by permission of Dedalus Press, www.dedalus.com.

Peter Kane Dufault, 'Evensong', from *Looking in All Directions*, Worple Press, 2000. Used by permission of Worple Press.

Carol Ann Duffy, 'Prayer', from *Mean Time*, Anvil Press Poetry, 1993. Used by permission of Anvil Press.

T. S. Eliot, 'Little Gidding', from *Collected Poems*, Faber and Faber, 1974. Used by permission of Faber and Faber Ltd.

D. J. Enright, 'Memory', from *Old Men and Comets*, Oxford University Press, 1993. Used by permission of Oxford University Press.

U. A. Fanthorpe, 'BC/AD', from *Standing To*, Peterloo Press, 1982. Used by permission of Peterloo Press.

Christopher Fry, from *A Yard of Sun*, Oxford University Press, 1970. Used by permission of Oxford University Press.

John Heath-Stubbs, 'Homage to J. S. Bach', from *Selected Poems*, Carcanet, 1990. Used by permission of David Higham Associates.

Anthony Hecht, 'Peripateia', from *Millions of Strange Shadows*, Oxford University Press/Athenaeum, 1977. Used by permission of Oxford University Press.

Zbigniew Herbert, *Report from the Besieged City*, Oxford University Press, 1985. Used by permission of Oxford University Press.

D. H. Lawrence, 'There is nothing to see', from *Complete Poems*, Penguin, 1993. Used by permission of Pollinger Ltd.

Jamie McKendrick, 'Give or Take', from *Ink Stone*, Faber and Faber, 2003. Used by permission of Faber and Faber Ltd.

Alice Meynell, 'The Unknown God', from *The Poems of Alice Meynell*, Burns, Oates and Washbourne, 1924. Reproduced by kind permission of The Continuum International Publishing Group.

Sally Purcell, 'Poem for Lent or Advent', from *Sally Purcell: Collected Poems*, Anvil Press Poetry, 2002. Used by permission of Anvil Press.

Rainer Maria Rilke, 'Book of Hours' 1,19, from *Rilke's Book of Hours: Love Poems to God*, Penguin Riverhead, 1996. Used by permission of Janklow and Nesbit Associates.

—*Duino Elegies VIII*, published by Chatto & Windus, reprinted by permission of The Random House Group Ltd.

R. S. Thomas, 'Suddenly', from *Collected Poems 1945–1990*, Phoenix Press, 2000. Used by permission of Phoenix Press, a division of The Orion Publishing Group.

W. B. Yeats, 'The Municipal Gallery Revisited VII' and 'A Prayer for Old Age' from *Collected Poems*, Dent, 1992. Used by permission of the Curator of the Works of W. B. Yeats, University of Dublin.

Every effort has been made to obtain permission for extracts from copyright material; the publisher apologises for any omissions and would be happy to rectify these in future reprints.

INTRODUCTION

Pressed by my editor to write another book, I stood firm. I was confident that four books were more than enough: everything I had it within my power to say had been said. Only a certain amount of what is rumbling around in our heads is worth sharing, and there is only a limited number of ways of rehearsing the same material without becoming tiresomely repetitive. And besides, my last book (*Learning to Dance*) was very much a *final* book, the last chapter, on the need to let go in old age and the reality of death, intended as a signing-off.

So much for predicting your own future. Never say never. For, just as M.E. (myalgic encephalomyelitis) had come along 20 years ago and hit me in mid-flow, knocked me flat and changed my life, so in the summer of 2005 cancer of the jaw came along and once again sent me spinning. From that icy moment of diagnosis, when you know that everything has changed, I recognised two things. First, that this would prove an unwanted but important test of the integrity of what I most deeply believed, both as a human being and a priest: a kind of inquest on all those words spilled out of pulpits or in counselling others or at hospital bedsides. A few months earlier I had attempted to tease out what I had come to think of as 'the enduring melody' of my life. This was the time to see how well it would stand up to the fiercest scrutiny.

Secondly, I felt the need in whatever lay ahead not to waste the experience, but to write about it as honestly as I could day by day, both as a form of therapy and (hopefully) to bring something creative and redemptive out of an inevitably dark time.

When, 20 years ago, I wrote *A Year Lost and Found* about the whole experience of M.E., it was before much was known about it. It had not yet been confirmed by the British Medical Association as an organic illness, but had been too often casually dismissed as 'yuppie 'flu'. When the book appeared, I was asked by an elderly, deeply pastoral priest if I enjoyed 'undressing in public'. I admired him for being a perfect example of a particular kind of English reticence, admirable in its way, that thinks it bad form to speak too personally of one's inner life and feelings, or to admit to those times of vulnerability and lack of confidence that we all recognise as part of our human journey. A form of self-indulgence. This can be complicated by the fact that many professional people – priests, doctors, teachers, lawyers – are wary of letting down their defences, except sometimes among their own kind, but even here most clergy are pretty cagey and defensive. And sometimes such wariness is a necessary safeguard for the well-being of patients, clients, pupils or parishioners. Counsellors and advisers must keep their distance. It's a fine judgement to have to make. But such reticence comes at a cost, that of seeming to cut ourselves off from sharing a common human experience that can make the journey that bit less lonely and help authenticate perfectly normal, valid feelings (not least in finding the hint of a meaning in what feels meaningless) when we walk in the shadowlands of illness, pain or grief.

The response to that small book took me by storm. It sold nearly 15,000 copies and led to a flood of letters that proved almost overwhelming when I had moved on and had another busy life to live. Even now they sometimes still drop through the letterbox. It taught me that there is a different country which we enter when we suffer, and that those who have learned to feel their way through different forms of darkness, and spent time – for whatever reason – treading its paths, recognise each other and are more likely to turn to those who have been there too. The gift of empathy is all the better for being hard-won.

What follows in the major part of this book is my attempt
to write an honest account of what Mother Mary John of the
Benedictine community at West Malling described to me as
'the questioning country of cancer'. Cancer is unlike any
other illness which may attack the body in that, faced by
disease, by bacteria, viruses and toxins which are external
threats to the body, the body at once takes appropriate
counter-measures against them. But not cancer. The cancer-
cell is one that has up till now devoted itself to serving the
body; now it seems to 'change its mind', and instead of
serving the organ in question (and hence the greater
organism of the body), it makes its own reproduction its
primary aim and starts acting, not as a member of a multi-
cellular team, but regresses to the more primitive single-cell
organism. Then, thanks to the process of cell division, it
starts feeding on other cells and can spread steadily and
ruthlessly. Richard Dawkins famously wrote of 'the selfish
gene': this is 'the selfish cell', its ultimate purpose the
destruction of the host body, and therefore – paradoxically –
its own destruction as well. Unless it can be stopped. The
greater part of this book, then, is the record of the profes-
sionals' attempt to abort the cancerous cells at a relatively
early stage, and what that process felt like. It is a kind of
journal written daily as it happened and shows how vulnerable we all are, how fragile and unpredictable our hold
on life can sometimes be, and how miraculous is the skill of
twenty-first-century surgery; and it seeks to discover how far
'the melody' of faith endures. It is printed largely as written,
though I've cut out certain details that would have proved
tiresome.

What transforms such a time is having someone beside
you with whom you can share the journey, but it's easy to
downplay the cost to them. Theirs is a more difficult role,
requiring at times a deeply demanding patience and courage, and Alison has written about the days when I was in the
operating theatre and intensive care. Our children, Sarah (a
community nurse in Berkshire) and Mark (a deputy head of

a large comprehensive school in London), have written briefly about that time too, as have Sarah's children, 15-year-old Adam and 12-year-old Anna, who bravely came to see me in intensive care, when I looked not unlike the Elephant Man, before they left for a long-planned holiday in Eastern Europe. And my consultant surgeon, Ian Downie, has contributed a note about the surgical challenge he faced and its outcome. I'm grateful to them all. As I am to members of the local cancer care team, which embraces Southampton and Salisbury, and which cannot be faulted. A part of the NHS of which to be very proud.

The first two Parts were written with no thought of publication; but in the words of John Keats: 'Nothing ever becomes real until it is experienced.' Part I is my attempt to spell out (to use a musical analogy) my *cantus firmus*, the firm ground of a melody that has been shaped and refined over the years and which up until now has proved valid and enduring. In Part II I seek to set this in the context of ageing and the life of the spirit, to explore how things shift and resettle as you gently (or not so gently) slip into old age. Part III of this rather mongrellish book is the journal I kept during seven traumatic months after the cancer had struck, and by implication it asks if the experience affected what I had set out earlier. It is somewhat kaleidoscopic, the subjects shifting with my changing moods and not in as logical a sequence as they might be, so that I return to reflect on certain subjects – the nature of God, the power of words – from time to time. I know that there may be a few repetitions from previous books. This isn't deliberate, rather inevitable, and I ask you (if you have read any of them) to put it down to more than a touch of amnesia.

I'm only too aware of the dangers inherent in such a very personal book, particularly in the cancer journal. In a time of sickness your whole world contracts. Inevitably your concerns become fixed on your illness as you crawl through the slow process of biopsies, diagnosis and decisions about where and when the operation should be, and the anticipation and anxiety that creep up on you in the small, wakeful hours of the night; and soon your world is reduced even further to the four walls of the ward or the curtains around your hospital bed. In these circumstances it would be unnatural not to become self-centred, acutely conscious of every small change in your body; and self-concern is a near neighbour of self-indulgence. Some may find such detail superfluous; yet I've included it because it was the descriptions in *A Year Lost and Found* of what M.E. *felt* like that seemed to help people authenticate their own experience. In such writing the pronoun 'I' occurs with wearisome frequency. In an attempt to avoid this, R. S. Thomas, in his *Autobiographies*, uses the word Nemo ('Nobody') of himself, and the fifteenth-century mystic Margery Kempe tried substituting 'This creature' in place of 'I' and 'me'; but after a while the impersonal effect they are seeking is even more tiresome. And one's use of 'one' merely sounds pompous. Apart from my two chief consultants I have used initials for the professional medical staff of doctors and nurses.

I have tried not to make this a self-indulgent book. Yet I believe that a time of such an inescapable focus on yourself and your inner resources makes you more deeply aware of your fragile humanity; and if you desire it enough, it may make you more aware of what others endure daily, and deepen your empathy. In short, it can help stir up in you that most Christlike (and so Godlike) of gifts: the 'suffering alongside' another that stands at the heart of the Incarnation and which – since William Tyndale invented the word in his first English Bible – we call 'compassion'.

In *Adam Bede*, George Eliot writes of the redeeming of pain:

> It would be a poor result of all our anguish and our wrestling if we won nothing but our old selves at the end of it – if we could return to the same blind loves, the same self-confident blame, the same light thoughts of human suffering ... Let us rather be thankful that our sorrow lives in us as an indestructible source,

only changing its form, as forces do, and passing from pain into sympathy – the one poor word which includes our best insights and our best love.[1]

The novelist Ian McEwan, in an interview a few days after the collapse of the Twin Towers on 9/11, said this:

If the hijackers had been able to imagine themselves into the thoughts and feelings of the passengers, they would have been unable to proceed … Imagining what it is like to be someone other than yourself is at the core of our humanity. It is the essence of compassion and the beginning of morality.[2]

And in an interview on the following Sunday he said that novels are about

showing the possibility of what it is like to be someone else. It is the basis of all sympathy, empathy and compassion. Other people are as alive as you are. Cruelty is a failure of imagination.[3]

Only human beings have the power to imagine a future that could be different from the present; only we can begin to imagine what it might be like to be someone else. I believe that one of the ways in which God can use our experience of darkness is to increase our imaginative understanding, reaching out to one another with love because we have been there too.

PART I

The Cantus Firmus

'I mean,' protested the housekeeper, 'didn't any-body bother with your religious education? You do believe in *something*, don't you?'

Miss Hare hesitated. Then she said, very slowly: 'I believe ... I believe in what I see and what I cannot see. I believe in a thunderstorm, and wet grass, patches of light, and stillness. There is such a vari-ety of good. On earth. And everywhere.'

'But what is *over* it?' Mrs Jolley had to burst out.

'That!' Miss Hare cried. 'That! I would rather you did not ask me about such things.'

Patrick White[1]

Pin your faith on the *cantus firmus*.

Dietrich Bonhoeffer[2]

I was launched as a pale young curate into a church and a society which were almost unimaginably different from our own. It was the year after Suez; Harold Macmillan was Prime Minister; Gatwick Airport opened, as did *My Fair Lady* at Drury Lane. CND was launched, and the BBC Third Pro-gramme, and the state pension was raised to £2.50 a week. My annual salary was £330. Satire had not been invented. No one had heard of the Beatles. Rowan Williams was at primary school. Synods were not even a gleam in an arch-deacon's eye. The Church of England, under the head-masterly Geoffrey Fisher, sailed on, unaware of the distant icebergs of *Honest to God* and the so-called 'death of God'; not expecting the cultural revolution of the 1960s, unin-terested in questions of gender and sexuality, not yet having digested the words 'post-modern' and 'multi-faith'. A gen-erally respectful and sympathetic press kept its distance. People attended Evensong. Anglicans (a bit tentatively and somewhat patronisingly) dipped their toes in the waters of a different tradition once a year in the Week of Prayer for Christian Unity. We were, you might say, a fairly compla-cent lot. There have been many unwelcome, destructive changes since then, but it's not my purpose to spell them out. There are already too many prophets of doom and gloom. But rather, I want to thank God that so many of the changes of my lifetime have been wise, just and life-enhancing: a free health service; advances in medical tech-niques and skill, such as non-invasive surgery; more humane treatment of the disabled and the mentally ill; the advances in palliative care and – with a new understanding of the needs of the dying – the growth of hospices; the end of capital punishment; international aid agencies; laws affirming human rights; the beginning of concerted action against poverty and to protect the environment; an increasingly less class-ridden society; and (certainly among the young) a concern for justice for the poor and marginalised.

For both Church and State there have been radical shifts in our understanding of human sexuality, new ethical challenges raised by the power of medical technology, not least the potential for genetic manipulation, and the waning and rising of major ideologies affecting the power-structures of the world. For the Church of England, leaner now than then, there have been new, challenging insights into the role of women; new and far better forms of liturgy than its critics would allow; a broader concept of spirituality; and a more democratic way of making appointments. When we are not dismissed by the media as irrelevant, we are mocked for seeming to live in a world of fairy-tale. (Which, in the more extreme expressions of the faith, we surely do.) We are largely ignored by a society (76.9 per cent of whom still claim, for the purposes of the census, to believe in God; 71.6 per cent in some form of Christianity) which nevertheless has little time for figures to whom they once deferred, whether they be princes, bishops or politicians. We are demoralised by what feels like shifting ground in matters of belief, which has in some quarters led to an unattractive closing of ranks. We seem unsure of how to speak in an ambience of easy-come, easy-go morality without sounding negative and judgemental; and too often we find ourselves defending a church that is unbalanced by the over-emphasis on management and administration that has infected society as a whole; a church, moreover, somewhat obsessed by issues which often seem of borderline relevance to the Kingdom of God.

'The church,' said the former Archbishop of Canterbury, Robert Runcie, 'is like a swimming-pool: all the splashing goes on at the shallow end.' So what is it like at the deep end of the swimming-pool? We may be out of our depth (we trade, after all, in mystery), but is there some definable spiritual hinterland that does not change with passing fashion? I can only try to define what for me, after 49 years of a wonderfully varied ministry, has been and remains (and I believe will remain) constant, immutable and authentic. What I'm seeking is what musicians call the '*cantus firmus*', the firm ground, the absolute rather than the relative, learning to hold firm to the heart of the matter and sit light to the rest.

For most of the Middle Ages, church music consisted of the so-called Gregorian chant: one line of melody attached to the words of the liturgy, and until the ninth century that melody was left unclothed. That plainsong melody is the *cantus firmus*, the 'fixed song'. By the twelfth century it was found that two or more melodies could be combined, and the *cantus firmus* becomes the basis of a *polyphonic* composition through the addition of counterpoint. Gradually, the traditional plainsong, formerly sung in unison, began to be given to the singers of the middle voice – that is, the tenors (from the Latin *tenere*, to hold), literally the *holders* of the fixed song or the *cantus firmus* – while the higher and lower voices enwrapped it with the developing counterpoint. In the next three centuries the original melody was increasingly embellished by the *harmony* which clothes it and is built round it, offering the listener a melody visualised as being on top, and having 'below' a group of notes (a chord) that will please the ear. In the sixteenth century the two musical styles, the polyphonic and the harmonic, were combined by masters such as William Byrd, who introduced new subtleties of feeling in matching the words to the emotions. Byrd wrote:

> There is a certain hidden power in the thoughts underlying the words themselves, so that as one meditates and constantly and seriously considers them, the right notes in some inexplicable fashion suggest themselves spontaneously.[3]

Bach is the past master in the use of the *cantus firmus*. His *fugues* are built on a structure of a melody in the home key, the *cantus firmus*, which he then decorates, turns upside down, plays with, but always comes back to in the end. An Eastern Orthodox theologian writes:

> In Bach's music ... the potential boundlessness of thematic development becomes manifest: how a theme can unfold inexorably through difference, while remaining continuous in each moment of repetition, upon a potentially infinite surface of varied repetition ... In Bach's music, motion is absolute ... each note an unforced, unnecessary, and yet wholly fitting supplement, even when the fittingness is deferred across massive dissonances by way of the most intricate contrapuntal mediations ...[4]

4

There is both perfect order and infinite variety. So, in the *Goldberg Variations*, a simple aria is stated, which is then displaced by an amazing sequence of 30 variations composed not upon it, but upon the bass line, the *cantus firmus* 'in which every third variation is a perfect canon'. At the end the aria is restated, but now you hear it with new ears, for it has become richer for all the variations that have been played upon it. Again, at the end of Bach's unaccompanied *Violin Partita*, where the *cantus firmus* is a bass phrase of absolute simplicity four bars long, it is then restated in 64 variations which arrive at 'a restatement that contains all the motion, variety and grandeur of what has gone before'.

The poet John Heath-Stubbs, in his 'Homage to J. S. Bach', writes of how Handel is much lauded for his 'magnificent wings of melody,/ Setting the water of the Thames on fire with gold,' so that for those singing Handel's praises

> Old Bach's music did not seem to the point:
> He groped in the Gothic vaults of polyphony,
> Labouring pedantic miracles of counterpoint.
> They did not know that the order of eternity
> Transfiguring the order of the Age of Reason,
> The timeless accents of super-celestial harmonies,
> Filtered into time through that stupendous brain ...[5]

A challenging modern example of the *cantus firmus* is the *Veni Creator* (*Come Holy Spirit*), an anthem for Pentecost by the composer Jonathan Harvey. It starts with the melody being chanted by a baritone soloist, and Harvey then introduces fragments of the tune sung by different voices, before an unpredictable sequence (representing the multitude of tongues at Pentecost) gives the altos, tenors and basses the option of *choosing their own note-lengths*. This results in an extraordinary cacophony, which nevertheless is held together by the soaring sopranos singing the tune in unison; and the work ends with the whole choir singing together: 'Praise to thy eternal merit! Father, Son and Holy Spirit!' No one performance is ever quite the same, but the *cantus firmus* – that first baritone solo – is the rock on which the whole work is built.

I believe that the creation is an endless sequence of variations on the unchanging theme of God's creative love, and that the story of evolution reveals how life has developed (and is still developing) from its first primeval molecules into more and more profuse and elaborate complex forms. I believe that the give and take of love which lies at the heart of our universe (because it lies at the heart of what we mean by the Trinity) is the ground bass which we are invited to discover for ourselves. Freedom, the only condition in which love can act, has to be part of the deal. I am free to embellish my life in my own way: indeed, I am in part (but only in part) programmed by my DNA and upbringing to do just that. Which means that disorder and disharmony are only too evident. My life, like everyone else's, is a complex mixture of harmony and dissonance, but it is uniquely mine. Perhaps it is only as we grow old that we can discern the *cantus firmus* of which we can say: 'This has been mine and mine alone: however much I have deviated from it and chosen my own note-lengths, this is its ground bass. There are certain critical truths and experiences that have seized and shaped me, and it is this firm ground that speaks to me of what is authentic (and therefore authoritative), and to which I can return, touching base as it were, at every stage of my unpredictable human journey.'

I see this *cantus firmus* as having three strands. The *first* and most obvious (if we're lucky) is the great affirming relationships of human love and friendship. They provide the firm ground that enables you to glimpse the even deeper truth that, in the words of the Abbé Henri de Tourville: 'We are loved by God more than we can conceive or understand.' The *second* strand of our *cantus firmus* comes for many of us from experiences of beauty and order which we discover in the natural world, together with that deeper appreciation of what it means to be human which we absorb from the arts: from the way our spirits are fed by certain music, paintings, novels, poems, plays, films and spaces. The pictures that silence us, and in a sense judge us; those books in which we become absorbed and which continue to live in us long after they are finished; the drama that sends us out of the theatre a little wiser and more aware of our shared humanity; those buildings that give us a momentary sense of the transcendent; that music that seems to exist somewhere between matter and spirit. And the *third* strand, undergirding the whole, has to do with those ultimate existential questions that come under the general heading of 'faith'. Life offers us the possibility of claiming these three life-changing gifts: the experience of love and friendship; recurring experiences of beauty and order; and a few undeniable experiences of transcendence in our search for our elusive God, if we are prepared to give attention to the one who is the source of our lives, and discern his presence both in people and in his creation.

For me the *cantus firmus* has included not simply a vague concept of the transcendent, but that of the incarnate and affirming God: the Christlike God of the Word made flesh. On the eve of my ordination I read Dietrich Bonhoeffer's *Letters and Papers from Prison*. Not long before he was executed by the Nazis, Bonhoeffer wrote these words to a close friend:

> God requires that we should love him eternally with our whole hearts, yet not so as to compromise or diminish our earthly affections, but as a kind of *cantus firmus* to which the other melodies of life provide the counterpoint ... Where the ground bass is firm and clear, there is nothing to stop the counterpoint from being developed to the utmost of its limits ... Only a polyphony of this kind can give life a wholeness, and assure us that nothing can go wrong so long as the *cantus firmus* is kept going ... Put your faith in the *cantus firmus*.[6]

For Bonhoeffer, facing execution, it is the wholehearted love of God which is to be the ground bass, the firm ground, of his life.

7

I can only write of the form that the *cantus firmus* of faith takes for me: truths which lie not at the surface but at my deep centre, and which have been tempered and pruned over a lifetime. They have to do with words which, like all theological words, are hard to define with the precision the scientist demands: Incarnation and Eucharist; Cross and Passion; the nature of faith and the Kingdom of God. I will tease them out further in Part III.

My faith, that frame of mind which lies somewhere on the map which charts the territory between doubt and certainty, has not come wrapped in any neatly tied package. For all of us there will have been periods when God seems absent, but also moments, however rare, when, in the words of R. S. Thomas, God comes

> As I had always known
> he would come, unannounced,
> remarkable merely for the absence of clamour.[7]

For, in the words of John Donne:

> On a huge hill,
> Cragged and steep, Truth stands, and he that will
> Reach her, about must, and about must go.[8]

Faith is not about assenting to the truth of theological formulae. It's about a *relationship with God*, and like every living relationship, it has to be worked at, and the experiences of a lifetime will modify, refine and deepen it. My faith has been formed in me as I have reflected, and go on reflecting, on mystery. That's not a word much in favour with those unsympathetic to religious concepts. Contemporary observers see it as a cop-out. Yet the most humanist of scientists acknowledge how little we know about the universe or the human brain, and are not averse to using the word 'wonder'. There are mysteries which we cannot comprehend but which seem to comprehend us. 'Two things fill the mind', wrote Immanuel Kant, 'with ever new and increasing wonder and awe ... the starry heavens above me and the moral law within.'[9] But, as the poets and artists know, it's not just the starry heavens, for there is mystery in a blade of grass. My Christian faith has been formed in me as I have reflected on the mystery of Jesus, who is a kind of self-portrait of God in human terms and who, in claiming that God's name is Father and his nature is love, reveals all I need to know of the One whose creative Spirit holds me in being from moment to moment. In the words of the extended Preface from the eucharistic prayer for Christmas in *Common Worship*:

> In this mystery of the Word made flesh you have caused his light to shine in our hearts, to give knowledge of your glory in the face of Jesus Christ. In him we see God made visible and so are caught up in the love of the God we cannot see.

Or, in the words of John Donne:

> 'Twas much, that man was made like God before,
> But, that God should be made like man, much more.[10]

My faith has been formed in me as I have reflected on the mystery of the Cross and Passion, and Julian of Norwich's claim that 'love is their meaning'. And it goes on being formed in me as I continue to take my place within the community which is the Church, providing that I remember that the Church, for all its self-obsession, is simply the agent for the Kingdom, and that its task is not only to worship God, but to seek and celebrate signs of the Kingdom, wherever in the world they may be found.

Most of us, if we're lucky, can name one teacher who has transformed the way in which certain lifelong truths take their place in our lives. I had two. The second – the theologian – was my tutor at Cambridge, the chaplain of Corpus Christi, Roland Walls: wonderfully human and spiritual, mischievously funny, modest and wise and prophetic, one who loves the Church passionately (first as an Anglican, now as a Roman Catholic) but sees it in all its frequent absurdity. He is now in his nineties. He believes that religion has such a bad press because it has too often become a crusading ideology, creating division. Like Islam, Christianity has become involved with racism, class and nationalism.

> If the gospel can't get itself out of religion, in the sense of this imperial, triumphant, divisive stuff, then it's not going to be faithfully preached and proclaimed. If anybody asked me what is the purpose of my life as I see it now, I would say it's to contribute, in however small a way, to getting the gospel seen as transcendent to human religion.[11]

I can vividly remember sitting on Roland's sofa while he talked for an hour about the Kingdom: of how the Church was not to be identified with it:

> It's going to arrive. You're going to enter it. You're going to be invited to see it ... to be given it. In the Lord's Prayer we pray, 'Thy kingdom come,' together with its complementary twin request, 'thy will be done. Today. By us – but also, in spite of us.' By giving God space in my life.

So it means the rule of God, with all that implies. Justice, equity, honour, forgiveness, love.

So the Kingdom lies at the heart of the *cantus firmus*. And there are two further gifts: a corporate prayer and a corporate action. When the disciples ask Jesus to teach them how to pray, and a little later, when he shows them how he wants to be remembered, he gives them a dual *cantus firmus* which is universal and timeless. First, he gives them the Lord's Prayer. He provides them with a form of words which will form a deep bond of unity between them and among all Christians ever after – a kind of signature tune; and it contains all we will ever need to express our trusting relationship with God and our dependence on him. To say it slowly, in a thankful spirit, and conscious of the meaning that lies behind each word, is sufficient, even though unwrapping the layers of meaning in the words 'our' and 'Father' might take a lifetime. Yet no one has ever claimed that praying is easy. I may try to carve a few moments out of the day, or I may join others in worship, but very often my attention level is low, and at once the distractions come: all kinds of trivia (some of it very surprising) are washing round at the surface level of my mind and one thought leads to another, and I come to with a guilty jolt. And it doesn't improve with age. I take comfort from the fact that in our prayer life what matters is that a bit of me knows that there is within, *deeper than all the occasional doubts and constant distractions*, a *cantus firmus*, an awareness of and longing for the love of God as I have glimpsed it in those rare life-affirming moments (and will again). And I guess that's how it will continue to be, and that's all right, for my desire is to recall the melody, knowing at the deepest level that I am his, loved beyond my imagining and held by his grace.

But there is a second strand to the *cantus firmus* laid down by Jesus. For on that last night of his earthly life he gives them the shared meal of the Eucharist. And in it he spells out the four actions of taking, giving thanks, breaking and blessing which have been the four marks of his life, a *cantus firmus* for all who follow him and are prepared for their lives to be shaped in this same pattern. It has been called 'the body-language of God come into our midst'. Here is the pattern of self-giving love in a life *taken and offered back* to God, a life lived *thankfully*, a life *broken* and *shared* in the costly service of others. This is how we constantly touch base. 'Do this in remembrance of me.' The Greek word for 'remembrance' is *anamnesis*, not as simply a recalling of an action long buried in the past, but with the sense (in Dom Gregory Dix's words) of '"recalling" before God an event in the past so that it becomes here and now operative by its effects'.[12] This is how *we* are re-*member*ed, re-created, put together again as members of the Body of Christ; and therefore this is how *he* is re-membered in every sense and put together again, for he has no body now but ours, no hands to bless and heal, no voice to speak of the Father's love, but ours. This remembering (which is also a remembering) stretches across the world and backward and forward into time. For, whatever exact form the early *agapes* and Eucharists took, not a Sunday (and scarcely a day) has passed since that Last Supper when this pattern of his life has not been acted out by those who would be re-affirmed as members of his Body. In the words of Teilhard de Chardin, 'the incarnation realised in each individual, through the eucharist'.

When words and music are combined in a sung Eucharist, then the actions of taking, thanking, breaking and sharing are enriched in the unchanging *cantus firmus* of *kyrie*, *gloria*, *credo*, *sanctus*, *benedictus* and *agnus dei*. So the music of the *kyrie* can deepen our sense of penitence; that of the *gloria* our sense of wonder at God's grace; that of the *credo* our place in the worldwide Body of Christ; that of the *sanctus* and *benedictus* affirms our sense of God's holiness; and that of the *agnus dei* our need for the reconciliation of the Cross. Here music and worship fit together and enhance each other in a timeless pattern. The pattern chanted by monks all over Christendom during the first millennium; the music then codified in the early Middle Ages. This is the *cantus firmus* rising up to God somewhere in his world at every moment of the day and night. Every time the Lord's Prayer is said, each time the bread is broken and shared, people somewhere in the world are asking that the Kingdom may come on earth as it is in heaven. It is this steady and discernible melody of prayer and Eucharist, morning and evening, that is the ground bass of the Christian life, as constant as the tides advancing and receding on our seashores day after day after day. Something given, a sheer act of grace; and something given back in response, in obedience and trust.

It is difficult to understand how a few moments of intercession for Iraq or peace in the Middle East can be other than empty and ineffective words. No doubt they are often just that. But there is another possibility: that they are helping to redress the balance. That's a phrase which has come to mean more and more to me. *Redressing the balance*.

12

The daily papers and the nightly news are an incessant reminder that we live in a world, indeed a society, that is severely unbalanced. In the scales of justice, peace and human happiness, the balance seems heavily tipped in favour of injustice, suffering and violence. In human lives worldwide, pain and desolation, hunger and disease stalk the earth. And yet it would be a travesty of life not to place on the scales beside them the music of Beethoven and Mozart, the plays of Shakespeare and Chekhov, the novels of Tolstoy and George Eliot, the art of Rembrandt and van Eyck, the sculpture of Michelangelo and the poetry of Milton, George Herbert and Blake. (Those who dismiss such a list as 'elitist' should note the growth of theatres, not least 'fringe' theatres; the success of Classic FM, easy as it may be to mock its 'relaxing classics' at 2.00 and its 'smooth classics' at 7.00; the crowded art exhibitions; poetry in pubs; the burgeoning numbers of people signing up for classes in the arts and crafts.) And then there are the everyday experiences of loving and being loved, forgiving and being forgiven, the breathtaking beauty of the natural world, and the countless acts of compassion, courage, sheer human goodness and self-giving love, that are largely unreported but happen daily – what Wordsworth called 'the little nameless, unremembered acts/ Of kindness and of love'. The darkness is indeed very great, but not as powerful as the light, and even a single candle illuminates the dark. How, then, is the balance redressed?

Seamus Heaney calls one of his essays 'The Redress of Poetry', by which he means that it is the poet's task to act as a counterweight to the unbalance all about us, to redress the darkness by tilting the scales towards truths which are universal and transcendent. And George Steiner, in his autobiographical *Errata*, writes:

> In the midst of the inhumanity and indifference of history, a handful of men and women have been creatively possessed by the compelling splendour of the useless (the arts). It may be

that, together with the saints, secular and religious, they in some manner ransom mankind.[13]

In Heaney's phrase, poetry can offer a 'glimpsed alternative', a revealing of a way of seeing and understanding human life and human relationships which is constantly denied or threatened. Wilfred Owen, for example, by his refusal to dehumanise the enemy in the First World War; or (during the Soviet era) Irina Ratushinskaya, by her witness to human values in poems smuggled out of her Siberian prison. In such cases, the redress of poetry becomes an exercise in that most enduring of the gifts of the spirit: hope.

The poet whose work Heaney then singles out as the best example of what he calls 'the redress of poetry' is George Herbert, whose tiny church of Bemerton is now part of my home-town of Salisbury. He sees Herbert's work as witnessing to the best and most enduring Anglican spirit: a balanced, tolerant, measured, honest account of what it feels like to be caught up in the eternal paradox of doubt and faith, sin and grace. Poetry which sought to redress, and has continued to redress, the two extremes of Puritan fundamentalism and Catholic authoritarianism. And Heaney's fellow-Irishman, Michael Longley, says that he writes poetry because he sees it as an 'important way for humanity to redeem itself'.

In Richard Eyre's fine production of *The Merchant of Venice* at the National Theatre a few years ago, in the court scene in which Ian Holm as Shylock demands his pound of flesh, he enters with a pair of scales, which he positions centrally and sets up with great care; he then places in one of the dishes a pound weight. He whets his knife as he prepares with relish to cut the flesh from Antonio's chest and place it in the other dish to redress the balance. Portia pleads that he will have mercy, but he is resolute. With Shylock's knife about to cut into the flesh, Portia halts him with the warning that the pound must be exact, that if he allows one drop of Christian blood to spill he will pay the forfeit. Stunned, knowing himself defeated, Shylock asks leave to go, but Antonio demands that he is given half his possessions, and that at Shylock's death the other half will go to his cast-off daughter and hated son-in-law. He then adds, in a cruel act of revenge, that Shylock shall become a Christian. The Duke, who is judging the case, validates this. The Jew slowly takes off his *kippa* (skull-cap), prayer-belt and apron, holds them in the air and, his eyes meeting Antonio's mocking gaze, drops them in the scales' empty dish. They outweigh the pound weight and the dish tips down. The silence is held; his eyes don't leave Antonio's face; the point is made. Then Shylock shuffles off stage, his identity destroyed, a broken man. For all his lack of human feeling and sense of ven- geance, Shylock has revealed the hypocrisy of the equally unmerciful Christians. If Antonio's hatred and vicious anti- Semitism could have changed into some resemblance of the Jewish virtue of mercy, that alone would have redressed the balance. As it is, Antonio proves as murderous as Shylock, unlike the Duke in his treatment of the hypocritical Angelo at the end of *Measure for Measure*, or Hermione faced with the jealous Leontes in *The Winter's Tale*, where the balance is redressed by the liberating power of forgiveness.

But I'm not concerned here with poetry or drama, but with what may be called 'the redress of Christianity' in daily life. It, too, offers a 'glimpsed alternative', a way of seeing and understanding human life and relationships when they seem to be denied or threatened by the darkness. And I see the 'glimpsed alternatives' of prayer and Eucharist as being two most potent instruments in redressing the balance and helping to tip the scales of justice. When we meet together to break and share bread, where all kneel side by side and receive – as it were – of the same loaf, then we are acting out in miniature what God desires for his creation. It is, in its own small and local way, a fleeting but true foretaste of the longed-for universality of the Kingdom. Moreover, we are taking the products of the earth and doing with them what is intended: offering them back to their Creator thankfully, and sharing them equally. Each Eucharist, whatever else it may be, is a sign of our desire to redress the balance. In the same way, prayer is the way in which we turn aside, however briefly, to give attention to God, to become aware of who we are and whose we are; and when we intercede for others, we are redressing the balance by rejecting the world's assumption that we must each fight our own corner, and affirming that we are indeed members one of another; that loving God implies loving my neighbour as I love myself. In the words of Karl Barth: 'To raise the hands in prayer is the beginning of an uprising against the disorder of the world.'

These days I groan inwardly when people ask me: 'Is there a future for the Church of England?' as if expecting the answer 'no', and as if retirement confers on you singular gifts of prophecy. None of us can know what shape the church may take in the coming years. All I know is that prayer and Eucharist and the community they create will continue to lie at its heart, and that people will not cease to be in need of love and affirmation. Whatever form 'being church' may take, however new generations of Christians may embellish the *cantus firmus* of faith, it is inconceivable that worship and sacrament and pastoral care will not be part of that firm ground. They have proved authentic for two millennia and – however they may need to be expressed in changing times – they will, I believe, be equally valid for generations to come.

But I come back in the end to that truth which stands behind, before, under and over our prayer and worship, and all our actions as Christian communities. One that creates afresh the *cantus firmus* in every generation and sustains those who put their faith in it. And that is the mystery of Jesus, the human image of the invisible God, whose spirit could not be confined to a tomb, but is encountered in the most unexpected people and the most surprising places. In the end, to be a Christian is to opt to live your life in the light of your relationship with the God revealed in Jesus Christ. J. B. Lightfoot, one-time Bishop of Durham, wrote to his lifelong friend, Archbishop Benson, a week before his death: 'I find that my faith suffers nothing by leaving a thousand questions open, so long as I am convinced of two or three main lines'; much as the great historian, Herbert Butterfield, ended his *magnum opus, Christianity and History*, with the words: 'Hold to Christ and for the rest be totally uncommitted.' And a hundred years ago, George Tyrrell, the Roman Catholic priest whose modernist views finally led to his excommunication, wrote of the evening office *Tenebrae*, when all the candles are slowly extinguished except for the highest of all:

> As at Tenebrae, one after another the lights are extinguished, till one alone – and that the highest of all – is left, so it is often with the soul and her guiding stars. In our early days there are many – parents, teachers, friends, books, authorities – but, as life goes on, one by one they fail and leave us in deepening darkness, with an increasing sense of the mystery and inexplicability of all things, till at last none but the figure of Christ stands out luminous against the prevailing night.[14]

That solitary figure stands at the heart of my own *cantus firmus*. If the atheists are right and I am proved to be wrong; if my deepest beliefs are what many dismiss as mere fairytales; if there is nothing at the end but Prospero's 'such stuff/ As dreams are made on, and our little life/ Is rounded with a sleep'; then I shall still not wish to have lived in any other way, or to have based this one precious life on other facts and allowed them to define and motivate all I have done. For, despite all the darkness, they have not only brought much persisting joy, but I can think of nothing that would have so satisfied my deepest and most haunting human desires, convictions and hopes. I'm moved by, and share the words of R., one of our most original and perceptive friends, who cannot take the petty concerns and obsessions of the Church and yet 'would die for the point of it'.

To live in hope is not to live with a false sense of optimism. Nor is it only the old who are sometimes tempted to despair that the world seems to be governed by fury. The wells of peace are poisoned, the cries of the suffering largely ignored. On the day that the Twin Towers were demolished, an estimated 35,600 of the world's children died from conditions of starvation. Yet despair is never an option, and those who follow Christ need to hold in a fine balance two great requirements that our faith lays upon us. The first is that of love: love for the world in all its need, that together we may 'act justly, love mercy, and walk humbly with our God'. The second is to remember that there is a world elsewhere. The world is truly a place of oppression, poverty and disease, but that's only one half of the story. For the horrors of war and the violent acts of the wicked don't abolish beauty, destroy art, overthrow truth or nullify love and compassion. Yeats wrote of how no man can create like Shakespeare, Homer or Sophocles, 'who does not believe with all his blood and nerve, that man's soul is immortal'.

For years the writer Bernard Levin suffered from a severe form of Alzheimer's. He ended one of his last essays, on Christmas Eve 1992, with these words:

> The eternal verities are not changed, not even damaged, by the wickedness and the despair ... Provided that we do not try to deny the terrible reality, there is no shame in retreating to the Schubert quintet, to Shakespeare's *Sonnets*, to the *Rondanini Pieta* (of Michelangelo). Whatever Christmas means to us, from nothing to everything, it will last for ever. And love, the beloved republic, may weep, but will abide.[15]

For Christians, Levin's 'beloved republic' is a monarchy: it is the beloved Kingdom, where Christ reigns, with its great abiding and eternal verities: love, justice, mercy and truth.

And, if we desire it enough, they *will* abide.

PART II

The Time of Harvest

We live our lives for ever taking leave.
Rainer Maria Rilke[1]

When little is left of the flower
you revisit your roots.

D. J. Enright[2]

Let your last thinks all be thanks.

W. H. Auden[3]

The whole business of religion is gratitude.
Thomas Traherne

One Sunday night last year I invited Alan Bennett and
Patrick Garland to come to Salisbury Playhouse for a charity
performance in aid of the Medical Foundation for the Care
of Victims of Torture. They were presenting the life and
work of Philip Larkin, and Alan Bennett had given me the
title (from a Larkin poem) of *Down Cemetery Road*. Weeks
later, the publicity having gone out, Patrick Garland con-
tacted me and said that Alan must have forgotten that,
fearing that the title was negative and off-putting, they had
changed it to a more supportingly positive line from another
Larkin poem, *An Enormous Yes!* Hopefully those two titles are

19

not as contradictory as they sound. If that Jewish rabbi is on the right lines in suggesting that at the final judgement the first question God will ask us is, 'Did you *enjoy* my creation?' and if we can answer 'yes', it will be because we have lived our lives with our eyes opened to all kinds of beauty, finding here much to delight us, despite the darkness and the pain. Perhaps, at the end of Cemetery Road, there really is an enormous divine 'Yes!' in which all our 'yesses' meet and are finally satisfied. Though Larkin would have dismissed the thought as sentimental nonsense.

But, whatever the unimaginable future, for the present we are caught up on this often rather messy journey called life. Bill Bryson begins his entertaining and comprehensive book, *A Short History of Nearly Everything*, with these words:

> Welcome. And congratulations. I am delighted that you could make it ... For you to be here now trillions of drifting atoms had somehow to assemble in an intricate and curiously obliging manner to create you ... For the next many years these tiny particles will uncomplainingly engage in all the billions of deft, co-operative efforts necessary to keep you intact and let you experience the supremely agreeable but generally under-appreciated state known as life ... Being you is not a gratifying experience at the atomic level. For all their devoted attention, your atoms ... are mindless particles, and not even themselves alive. Indeed, it's an arresting notion that if you were to pick yourself apart with tweezers, one atom at a time, you would produce a mound of fine atomic dust, none of which had ever been alive, but all of which had once been you. Yet somehow for the period of your existence they will answer to a single rigid impulse: to keep you you. The bad news is that the atoms are fickle and their time of devotion is fleeting ... Even a long human life adds up to only about 650,000 hours. And when that modest milestone flashes into view, for reasons unknown your atoms will close you down, then silently disassemble and go off to be other things. And that's it for you.[4]

When it all started, this staggering creation, there were just two elements, hydrogen and helium, which were slowly transformed by the force of gravity, bonding together and forming stars. Those stars exploded. That created new atoms, and we are the waste, the stardust. And atoms can't be created or destroyed by anything scientists know how to do (though they can be split, with devastating effect). It is the same mix of atoms from the very beginning of time and for ever, and each one of us is made up of some 10,000 trillion trillion of them, but each put together in unique and elaborate ways, making complex molecules. Set on a tiny planet surrounded by Kant's 'starry heavens', which extend more than ten billion light years from us, and are expanding. To say nothing of the mysterious 'dark matter', which makes up 85 per cent of the universe, and still astronomers have no idea what it is.

One of the mixed blessings of being unique is that we're aware that at the heart of life there is an ultimately unbridgable aloneness. In the words of Job: 'Naked I came from my mother's womb, and naked I go back.' After the nine months lying close to our mother's heart, moving to her rhythms and warmed by her blood, we make that first journey from darkness into light alone; and finally, when the body is weary and worn out, we leave the light and go into the darkness alone. Even if we are surrounded by those who love and affirm us, and who enrich our human journey in a thousand different ways. This aloneness, proof of the precious gift of difference, is sometimes – though not necessarily – synonymous with loneliness. You can choose (and sometimes need) to be alone, but few would choose to be lonely. Aloneness may bring the pleasure of that solitude we all sometimes need, but isolation is unnatural, and it's just this recognition that we are ultimately alone which causes us instinctively to stretch out for the comfort of each other in our need for love. The American poet Anthony Hecht writes of the experience of sitting in a crowded theatre when the lights dim just before the play starts, 'and bring a stillness on':

    It is that stillness
I wait for.
    Before it comes,

Whether we like it or not, we are a crowd ...

But in that instant ...

Each of us is miraculously alone
In calm, invulnerable isolation,
Neither a neighbor nor a fellow but,
As at the beginning and end, a single soul,
With all the sweet and sour of loneliness.[5]

There will be times when we experience 'the sweet and sour of loneliness'. For although we share 99.9 per cent of our DNA, and are made up of the same kinds of cells and neurons; although we respond to kindness and cruelty, to the beauty of an English spring and the genius of Mozart or a Constable sky; although we are, like Shylock, 'fed with the same food, hurt with the same weapons, subject to the same diseases, healed by the same means, warmed and cooled by the same winter and summer'; and although all our stories share the same age-old themes of love and hate, ambition and jealousy and betrayal, courage and generosity, which enable us to feel for each other the precious gift of empathy; yet I am not you: I am *me*, uniquely me; and not even the one with whom I have shared my life knows *all* the secrets of my heart, nor I hers; or what it *feels* like to inhabit this skin and not another. And each of us experiences our own story as extraordinary, singular and worth the telling. When I walk in the country, read a novel, watch a film or play, look at paintings or listen to music, my response may be similar to yours, but it won't be exactly the same. When I am ill, it is my illness, my M.E., my cancer, and it takes on my particular characteristics. If I'm bereaved, my grieving may exhibit all the classic signs of anger, depression and self-pity, but my grief will be mine alone, for no one else begins to understand the nature of my love for the one I've lost, or can dare to say: 'I know what you're going through.' When I pray, I may follow patterns suggested by others, but I do so in my own unique way, and the familiar mixture of words and silence, good intentions and distracting thoughts, is mine alone. And when I say my prayers, my concept of the God I seek to address will not be quite the same as yours. And it is precisely this difference, the fact that no one else in the universe loves or laughs or grieves or prays or worships just like me, or ever will; it is this uniqueness, that makes us precious to one another and, I believe, uniquely precious to the God who must revel not in the sameness but in the infinite variety of his creation.

When I was a teenager, dressed in wartime black-out material stuffed with crunched-up newspapers, I stood on the stage of Torquay Town Hall with three other prunes and sang a song about old age called 'The Prune Song':

No matter how young a prune may be,
he's always full of wrinkles;
we get wrinkles on our face,
prunes get 'em every place ...

It was not my finest hour. But now I see things from the prune's point of view. The question whether the trip 'down Cemetery Road' is to be thought of as 'downhill' or 'uphill' depends, no doubt, on whether you are at heart a pessimist or an optimist.

Going uphill is much harder, but there may be a worthwhile view at the top. The thought of going downhill, while it may reflect an inevitable physical and mental decline, seems to deny that the constructive way to respond to every stage of life is with a 'yes', drawing upon a lifelong balance of good. In trying to assess the gains and losses of old age, we all hope that the decline will be mercifully gradual, but for many it won't. In one sense the decline of our mental powers begins when our brain cells start dying after we have peaked in our early twenties. It starts getting gradually more noticeable as we freewheel through our sixties and seventies

– though that may not be true for babies being born within our children's lifetime with a life expectancy of 100, and some scientists are predicting even longer life-spans as they gain mastery in the field of genetics and ever-more-effective control of mortal diseases. Not entirely a cheerful thought. Then things begin to accelerate: an illness or an accident knocks us back further than it once would have done; stiles are more challenging; bits of well-worn hips and spines wear out; once-familiar names resist recall; you wander into rooms and forget what you've come for. Our reflexes slow down, especially when driving. One of the hardest battles I ever had with my age-defying mother was to persuade her to give up her car at the age of 90. Luckily the law was on my side, for she had driven through Torquay's pedestrian precincts so many times 'because it's the quickest route to the doctor' that the police threatened to take her to court if she didn't see sense and relinquish her licence. Here, our car lives in the road outside our terrace house. Not long ago I went and cleaned it, feeling pleased with its new shine. 'Great,' said my wife when I pointed it out, 'but that's not actually our car.' Same make, same colour, and one satisfied but perplexed neighbour. 'The time will come in your life', writes John Mortimer, 'it will almost certainly come, when the voice of God will thunder at you from a cloud: "From this day forth thou shalt not be able to put on thine own socks." '[6] But along with our laughter at how absurd we are becoming, there is the shadow of a deeper anxiety that signals a real apprehension of what may be to come.

There are the social diminishments, such as the challenge of retirement from a job or a role where many have depended on your skills to one in which you are no longer in charge and will come increasingly to depend on others. Or having to meet common reactions to the old: being patronised, or not being noticed at all. ('You're standing in my light,' said a sort of Barbie doll to me recently when we came face-to-face on a narrow path, and I spent the rest of the walk thinking up things I might have said if my reflexes were sharper and if she hadn't been accompanied by two large youths.) It's difficult to come to terms with change, not least for churchgoers who have been nourished by the incomparable language of the *Book of Common Prayer* and the King James Bible, and perhaps have learned by heart passages that become strong spiritual supports in old age, who must now grapple with new translations and new liturgies, and whose plea for the occasional comfort of the familiar is not always heard with much sympathy. There are the inevitable deaths of friends and contemporaries, fewer and fewer with whom to share memories; and often the loss of a life-partner, with all the grief and desperate loneliness that can bring: no longer is there someone beside you with whom to share and laugh about the small intimacies of every day. We try to remember the face in its different moods, the shape of lips, a touch; the way he listened, the way she laughed. 'Grief,' said the late Queen Mother, 'doesn't get any easier: you just get better at it.' And for some, there may be an increasing sense of being hemmed in and relegated to the margins, as their world narrows down, even perhaps to the four walls of a room in a residential home. And there may be, as part of this inevitable diminishment of the sense of self, also a sense of a loss of God and a questioning of those beliefs that have previously sustained you.

One of the undoubted spiritual classics of our time is W. H. Vanstone's *The Stature of Waiting*. We may, for reasons of sickness or the incapacity of old age, become powerless and vulnerable – those who, with Milton in his blindness, can only 'stand and wait'. Jesus may not have known those particular rigours, but Vanstone sees the Gospel accounts of his life as falling into two parts: a dynamic *activity*, and then (from the start of his Passion in the Garden of Gethsemane) a brief but intense *passivity* in which he is in the hands of others, totally dependent on what they do to him and what they do for him: he is treated as worthless, bound, imprisoned, mocked. He has to be helped to carry his own cross.

Vanstone takes this deepest of all mysteries, that of God revealing himself as one who knows what it is to be vulnerable and powerless, and links it to the pattern of our own lives as we grow old, increasingly becoming those who are no longer proactive but reactive, people who must learn to be waited on without resentment and with proper gratitude; to let go with grace. And not feel that we are of any less value as human beings.

But for some, ageing will bring a far more painful loss. Senile decay or Alzheimer's present challenges, especially for those closest to you, and raise difficult questions about what it means to retain our singular integrity, as year by year a bit more of us goes missing. The brain is still so little understood and there are some unaccountable mysteries: for instance, cases where musicians can still play or sing familiar music even when they have lost the power of rational speech. I think of P., a musician lying in a deep coma in intensive care. The lifeline on the machine monitoring his heartbeat was barely flickering. They played him a recording of his favourite piece of music, Mozart's *Clarinet Concerto*. By the end the line was much stronger, and a few hours later he emerged from his coma. The neurologist Oliver Sachs famously writes of an elderly musician who was unable to distinguish his wife from his hat. The only way he could get dressed to go for a walk was by humming a Schumann song whose melody he remembered perfectly, and somehow that residual memory enabled him correctly to identify the former from the latter.

The losses, however, need to be counterbalanced and redressed by the not-inconsiderable gains. I don't just mean bus passes, free television licences and senior citizens' morning matinées at the local Odeon (with free coffee and, on high days, a raffle), but not so easily listed, rather more subtle, gains. The big events that have shaped a life, the times both of darkness and light, become burned into the grain of who we are. If we're wise we shall have learned from them and gained new understanding of what it is to be human. Inevitably there will be regrets, and curiosity about the path not travelled – 'Where might I be now if I'd done this rather than that?' – and you see how your life has often turned on some seemingly trivial moment: a word said, a meeting, a saying 'yes' rather than 'no', or (more likely) 'no' rather than 'yes'. We may regret some of the things we did, and at the same time regret even more the things we hadn't the courage to tackle. In the words of William James which Thomas Hardy copied into his commonplace book, 'we live forward, we understand backward'; or, as Coleridge wrote: 'The light which experience gives is a lantern on the stern, which shines only on the waters behind us.'

There is a profound difference between those who view their lives *simply* in terms of Shakespeare's seven ages – from the infant 'mewling and puking in the nurse's arms', to that 'second childishness, mere oblivion,/ Sans teeth, sans eyes, sans taste, sans everything'[7] – and those who see their lives also as an *inner* journey, a journey of the spirit as we travel home to God. At first our journey is from dependence to a proper independence, the search for identity, meaning and self-worth, and coming to terms with our sexuality, growing in knowledge and experience. The second kind of journey, from independence to dependence, is different. The autumn of our lives is also the time for learning a new dependence on God, who in Isaiah says to his people:

> Listen to me ... (you) whom I have carried from the womb,
> whom I have supported since you were conceived.
> Until your old age I shall be the same,
> until your hair is grey I shall carry you.
> As I have done, so I shall support you ...[8]

It's also a time for learning new skills, things we've not previously had time for, learning to see not just the inevitable endings but also the potential beginnings. The ageing Prospero swears that from now on 'every third thought shall be my grave' which, comments the writer John Updike,

27

'leaves two other thoughts to entertain above the ground: love one another, and seize the day'. Loving one another doesn't get much easier with age, but perhaps 'seizing the day' does. For with an increasingly limited time ahead, I think of those places I shall never see, and those things I shall never do, and I come to see that it doesn't matter: that what alone matters is that I begin to come to terms with what I have made of my life in the only moment that counts, which is the moment that is 'now'. I try to say each morning, adapting the words of the Psalmist: 'This is the day which the Lord has made; this is the place where I must look for him; and those I meet today are the people whom the Lord has given: let me rejoice and be glad in them.'

There is another quality of old age that can be pure gain, and not just for ourselves: wisdom. Once people were called elders because in a long life they had harvested wisdom – which is very different from that gathering of information with which our culture is obsessed. Wisdom is not what you know about: it's what you *know*, deep inside you, the very essence of your inner life. Wisdom is the art of holding together the old and the new, of balancing the known with the unknown, the pain and the joy; it's a way of linking the whole of your life together in a needful integrity. 'Growing' ought to mean just that: growing as we age. Growing in a sense of wonder at the familiar and in curiosity about the new – just plain curiosity about life which, said Dr Johnson, is what most clearly demonstrates 'a generous and elevated mind'. (Dorothy Parker was asked by a friend how to put down a seriously ill cat. She answered, 'Try curiosity.') Growing in wisdom, patience and the contentment to move more and more from *doing* into that equally rewarding and much more important state of *being*, so that we may discern what matters and what doesn't. It will mean detachment and learning to let go, and it may indeed mean replacing a life of independence with one of increasing dependence on others. We can't prepare ourselves for birth: we can for death.

28

> There comes the supreme day, [wrote Montaigne] the day that
> is judge of all the rest. 'It is the day' (as Seneca says) 'that must
> judge all my past years.' I leave the fruit of my studies for death
> to taste. We shall see then whether my speeches come from my
> mouth or my heart.[9]

The way we grow old and prepare to meet our death will
surely confirm or deny the validity of what we have said in
our lives. Some will fight the ageing process: others, like
Prospero at the end of *The Tempest*, will learn to accept it as a
journey towards a letting go of some of the chains we may
have wound around ourselves for our protection and our
comfort.

But generalisations about ageing, like all other generalisations, are useless. Some people seem middle-aged in the
cradle, and there are those in their nineties whose relish for
life is as vivid as it was in their twenties. I only know what it
feels like for me to be 76: it feels like all my ages wrapped
into one. There is always a bit of me that still *feels* 10 years
old, or 21, or a young father holding his first-born child, for
there is within each of us this recognisable and unchanging
core. The daily miracle that I – or anything at all – exists still
has the power to astonish me, as does the natural world with
its constantly shifting patterns and changing light. No two
days are ever quite the same. Near the end of Marilynne
Robinson's fine novel, *Gilead*, the narrator (a priest) is writing to his young son, born to him in old age by his second,
much younger, wife. It is a kind of love-letter to life itself:
'Wherever you turn your eyes the world can shine like
transfiguration', he says. 'There are a thousand thousand
reasons to live this life, every one of them sufficient.'[10] Like
many people, as I grow old I become more and more aware
of the mystery of my 'self', and of the life that 'self', united
with other selves, has been enabled to live. I know about
cells and genetics: that I was once an embryo and then a
foetus; but I can't begin to grasp the fact that when I was
born there was potentially enough information capacity in

each cell of my body to fill some dozen copies of the *Encyclopaedia Britannica*, or that there are more cells in one of my fingers than there are people in the world. The more we discover about what it means to be an embodied spirit, the more we realise the hidden depths in the Psalmist's claim that we are 'fearfully and wonderfully made'.

Neurologists tell us that they understand about a tenth of what there is to know about the human brain, and are still baffled by the riddle of human consciousness; yet one of the most rewarding gifts of age can be to revisit the place where our vanished days are gathered: its name is memory. For many people, of course, memories may be largely painful and unrewarding; for some, agonisingly so. I'll come back to their negative aspect. But for most of us, it's the good memories of people which dominate, and those life-shaping events which remain as vivid as ever. 'Perhaps being old', wrote Philip Larkin, 'is having lighted rooms/ Inside your head, and people in them, acting.'[11] Old age ought to be the time when we can visit that place in order to better understand and integrate our lives, a time of harvest. 'You have sown so much', says the prophet Haggai, 'but harvested so little.' There's a poem by Jamie McKendrick called 'Give or Take':

> Just how heavy the human head is
> is easy indeed to underestimate.
>
> My sister tells me it weighs-in around
> 12 lbs, give or take a few fluid ounces
>
> of grey matter – she hands her pupils with back pains
> a shrunken headsized lethal *petanque*
>
> of pitted golden Cotswold stone
> that must have once adorned a balustrade
>
> before rolling off its stalk with an archaic thud
> and gets them to imagine walking round

with one of those balanced on their backbones
– and that's not even counting all the thoughts

which laid end to end would span the equator
and weigh as much as the world itself.[12]

Everything I have ever seen and every person with whom
I've spent time have somehow been translated by my brain
into images and feelings, and I can immediately conjure up
a host of them from that most strange yet intimate centre
that is 'me'. At the level of my unconscious all my experiences exist timelessly, for what we call 'time' is merely the
way we turn the flow of successive moments into some kind
of manageable order. When I seek to tell my unique story, it
is by linking together memory and imagination. For then I
can gather lost moments and experiences, overcome the gap
between past and present, bring them together and hold
them as one. This is how we gain a hold on truths which
seem to us timeless, and which speak of human experiences
that are universal. Which is why it can be so devastating
when memory fails. We are born, we grow, we are moulded
and changed by life; though sometimes, looking back, the
old 'me' may seem almost unrecognisable. The novelist
Graham Swift writes of a character looking at a photograph
of himself as a child; of how he stares at it and the child
returns his gaze 'as if from another world, another planet.
Was that really *me*?' And the child stares back 'as if he
doesn't know (me) either, has never seen (me) before in his
life'.[13]

And yet I can recognise a consistency in the responses and
the behaviour of my friends and loved ones, as they do in
mine. I am still unmistakably 'me'. I know that if I have a
sense of worth and integrity it's because I have been
affirmed over a lifetime in the give and take of love. My
body is ageing, but I am not just my body. My brain takes
longer to come up with facts, but I am not just my body plus
my brain. I am much more than the sum of my parts. And
yes, that child who stares out at me from the yellowing

photograph album really is me, and I still carry him within me. I recently went back to my school for a reunion lunch of all those who left before 1955. It was a mistake. Part of you goes on remembering school contemporaries as willowy youths, unscarred by life, not as bald and plump and deaf and (in some cases) rabidly right-wing. (Am *I* really like that? Increasingly 'yes' to two of the four.) Even so, I found I could say of those I remembered: 'We may not have met for nearly 60 years, but you are still recognisably you.' It is this singular flavour, this consistent identity, which makes each of us not only uniquely different but uniquely precious, both in the eyes of those who love us and also in the sight of God; and it is this mysterious integrity of our lives that can reassure us as we reflect on the known past and peer into the unknown future.

We each have our own story to tell, like and unlike everyone else's story. We each need to discern it and marvel at how, in retrospect, it begins to make sense, and we can see how everything – the bad times when God seemed to have deserted us as well as the good – was grist to the mill; and how, a bit battered, we have not only come through but (hopefully, though not always) learned lessons that make us more rounded people; how all in the end is part of the harvest of our lives. For those who are granted the grace of a reasonably healthy and unbefuddled old age, one of its gifts is the chance to explore the shape of one's life and its inner journey – all the relationships, all the experiences of beauty and sorrow, love and loss, all that we know to have been authentic and which has formed and changed us, and made us what we are. The temptation in old age is to say, 'I am what I *was*.' But that's only half the truth: until the day I die, I am what I *am*. And when I come to die, I shall no longer have a past. I shall be remembered as a complete being, formed by my relationships and by all that happened to me and what I made of it. For even now there is a consistency and a harmony about my whole life. Whether good or bad or indifferent, happy or unhappy or with spells of both, it hangs together. This uniqueness that is 'me' is what I have to offer to my Creator, who knows me infinitely better than I know myself, and graciously welcomes me home, not in spite of what I have been but because of what I am. 'Graciously': the action of grace. 'Home': the place where I can shed all pretence, where 'everything is known and yet forgiven'.

But what of the unfinished business, the unrighted wrongs, the negative memories that come back to haunt us in dreams or in the wakeful hours of the night? Central to achieving a gracious, contented old age is how we acknowledge the great healing power of forgiveness: forgiveness both of ourselves and of others. For nearly 20 years I was a trustee of St Christopher's Hospice. I learned so much there about the needs of the dying and their proper care. Its founder, Dame Cicely Saunders, and her vision and teaching, have been hugely influential in modern palliative care. At its best, such care is about enabling people to live as fully as possible until they die, surrounded by those who will provide the best possible medical and spiritual care, and ensuring, insofar as is humanly possible, that they have a good death. 'You matter because you are you, and you matter to the last moment of your life' has been Cicely Saunders' constant theme. While hospices have burgeoned in the 40 years since St Christopher's was founded as the first modern hospice, there are still too few of them, and patients who can receive first-rate palliative care – and increasingly this will be at home from Macmillan nurses – are still in a minority. But the lessons are beginning to be learned, not least in medical schools.

Cicely Saunders knew that when we come to die, we may experience two kinds of pain: physical pain, which in most cases can be effectively controlled by the expert use of modern drugs; and a less easily controlled spiritual pain (what she called 'soul pain'), where my very identity seems to be disintegrating and I need to be heard and reassured that my life has made sense and been of value. There may be all kinds of unsatisfactory loose ends – disappointments, family rows, anger, guilt, even bitterness – that need to surface and be resolved. At such times we may need above all else someone to sit beside us and listen as, in however stumbling a way, we tell our stories. In my local hospice, not only is art and music on the agenda, but once a week a small professional theatre company visits the day centre and allows the patients to talk about themselves, to remember people and events and find purpose and shape in their lives, and the company sometimes take away that material, dramatise parts of it, and go on to perform it in the wider community. In another hospice there has been the practice of using an artist to sit beside a patient and encourage him or her to describe in great detail one place which they love: perhaps a childhood home, or somewhere they have been deeply happy. The artist then goes away and draws or paints it, comes back and shows it to the patient, changes it until it seems right, and then gives it to the dying person to have beside them and make a last gift of it to whomever they wish.

But it shouldn't wait till then. For the chief task of the last period of my life (however short or long that may be) is a spiritual one: it is that of *integration*. Integration, in the life of a nation, a community, a family or an individual, is the art of bringing together what is scattered and diverse and forming a satisfying whole: its opposite is segregation, division, alienation. In personal terms, integration brings contentment and peace of mind, whereas the failure to integrate leads to discontent, depression and even despair. But we're complex creatures, and our minds function at a surface level, but also at a profoundly deep one as well. The surface mind, the home of the ego, is the 'me' that wants to be in control and fears the unknown, and needs the mask we all forge (consciously or unconsciously) with which to face the world. In childhood most of us learn to protect our vulnerability and bury deep all our unresolved baggage. This deep level is where we continue to store away unwanted thoughts and emotions, old hurts and painful memories. We may have carried a burden of hidden resentment or guilt. And one of the gifts of age is that we have the opportunity to lay these potentially damaging ghosts to rest. We may need help, but we can learn to address and settle our negative feelings, our wounds and our anger: facing, where it exists, the poison of resentment, to know ourselves forgiven, to accept that forgiveness and in our turn to forgive. Not only may we need to forgive others; we may need to forgive God or life itself; to exercise compassion, both for others and for ourselves; and at the same time, to seek to free ourselves from the understandable, but exhausting, need to possess, to achieve, to manipulate, to be the centre of attention.

Helen Luke, a Jungian analyst, was born in England, though she worked largely in the United States, founding there the Apple Tree Community. She is the author of a small book, *Old Age*, with the sub-title *Journey into Simplicity*,[14] and I'm indebted to her thoughts. She writes that it is as if, as we grow old, we have to learn a new language, what T. S. Eliot in 'Little Gidding' describes as 'the gifts reserved for age'. I've already touched on them. They are, first, the willingness to accept what the ego fights against: the gradual loss of energy, the diminishment of hearing or sight, the enforced move from active to passive. Secondly, we need to bring our nostalgia under control. Though the world of our youth may have been cruelly pushed into the past, its familiar touchstones – the songs, the clothes, the manners – are now considered quaint. We're not the first generation to feel (rightly or wrongly) that the change from then to now is largely for the worse, though it's never happened quite so fast. In Alan Bennett's *The History Boys*, Irwin comments that, 'There is no period so remote as the recent past';[15] and at the end of Chekhov's *Three Sisters*, Olga reflects that,

> Yes, we will be forgotten, such is our fate and we can't help it, and the things that strike us as so very serious and important,

35

they will be forgotten one day or won't seem to matter. The curious thing is we can't possibly know just what will be thought significant and important and what will seem pathetic or absurd.[16]

We may privately deplore the losses, but we must have the grace to celebrate the undoubted gains. And if the young won't listen to us, then that doesn't prevent us listening to – and maybe learning from – them, for they need hearing and affirming as much as we do, and we may find some of our prejudices challenged and even laid to rest.

But it's the *third* gift that is perhaps the hardest to accept. Either we continue, as we age, to cling to our past achievements, our desire to dominate and control, or we learn gracefully to let go and discover a new freedom and a new unity with the created world in all its beauty and its creatures in all their variety. We can begin to piece together the story of our lives; to look clear-eyed at the suffering and the sorrow hidden in our memories; to come to terms with our sins, our mistakes, our failure to love as we might have done, our desire (often unrecognised until now) to control and manipulate others. You might, then, call the three gifts the last stages of our physical, mental and spiritual development: *physical*, as we're called upon to face the fact of our failing senses; *mental*, as we become aware of the follies of our time, and accept our powerlessness to affect them; and finally, *spiritual*, as we suffer the remorse of reliving and coming to terms with some of our own past actions and motivation; where facing the darkness is an essential part of the healing, and which enables us to be restored by what Eliot calls the 'refining fire'. For him the 'refining fire' is God's awesome love and grace, and to experience it is to enter into the measure of the dance. 'At the still point of the turning world,/ At the still point, there the dance is.' The cosmic dance of Love.

As the Mock Turtle said to Alice: 'Will you, won't you, will you, won't you, will you join the dance?' As I grow old, it is this concept of the dance which becomes more and more important to me. The dance of creation: the dance of the laws of the universe to what was once believed to be 'the music of the spheres'; the dance of the planets in space and the dance of the molecules in my circulating blood and beating heart; the dance of the seasons and of the whole natural world and the tiniest particles of matter; the dance of faith in those painful times when it feels like dancing in the dark; and, best of all, the dance of relationships, of forgiveness and friendship and love, which have created the true and enduring melody of our lives. For Christians – certainly for Eliot – at the very heart of the dance is forgiveness and mercy, those qualities which translate as love. The point of integration that we search for all our lives, is that undergirding and affirming love to which we give the name of God.

In *Old Age* Helen Luke also considers two of Shakespeare's plays, *The Tempest* (his last) and *King Lear* (perhaps his greatest). All Shakespeare's final plays are about choice: a choice between justice and mercy, punishment and forgiveness, a choice so profound in its implications that it liberates and brings about change and transformation. The shipwrecked Prospero finds on his island Caliban and Ariel, and he is changed as he slowly learns to set them free. Luke sees them as the two aspects of our divided selves. As Prospero says of Caliban: 'This thing of darkness I acknowledge mine', and there is indeed a darkness within us that we need to face and come to terms with; but there is also an Ariel. Our discovery when young that we have certain inborn gifts and skills, which then come to maturity in our middle years, is the discovery of our own Ariel. Ariel is able 'to fly, to swim, to ride the curled clouds', and he is that creative, exploring, imaginative spirit that can enable us to lead creative and fulfilling lives. In the ageing Prospero, Shakespeare presents us with the choice which in the end we too have to face: whether to confront and so set free the ugly creature who is Caliban; and whether to cling tight to the graceful Ariel – or set him free as well. Because our thoughts about life become simpler and deeper as we age (fewer choices), we may be given the grace to understand that we have one overriding choice: to cling to our past achievements, growing resentful and lamenting what is lost; or to accept our natural loss of energy and growing weariness, feeding off our good memories of the past and laying to rest our bad ones. We can choose to reflect daily with thankfulness and wonder on this amazing gift of life, and so discover that in the end that letting go as gracefully as we can, however paradoxical it feels, is the measure of our gratitude for what we have been given.

Each heartbeat moves us a little nearer death. In Dante's lovely image: old age is like lowering your sails as you drift into harbour. In certain monastic communities it was once the practice to lie in your coffin as a way of meditating on your own mortality. A little extreme, we may think, a bit unEnglish. Yet meditating on our own death, and leaving clear instructions of the form we would wish our funeral to take, can be important for those who love you. The poet Charles Simic tells of his grandfather, who was diabetic, with one leg cut off at the knee and a strong chance of losing the other. Each day his friend Savo used to pay him a visit, when the two would reminisce about the past:

> One morning my grandmother was out attending a funeral. Simic's grandfather hopped out of bed and into the kitchen, where he found candles and matches. He got back into bed, somehow placed one candle above his head and the other at his feet, and lit them. Finally, he placed the sheet over his head and began to wait. When his friend knocked, there was no answer. The door was unlocked, so he came in, calling out from time to time. The kitchen was empty. Entering the bedroom, and seeing the candles, Savo let out a wail and then broke into sobs as he groped for a chair to sit down. 'Shut up, Savo!' my grandfather said sternly from under the sheet. 'Can't you see I'm just practising?'[17]

So we come full circle. When we were young, life seemed endless; now, we know how fleeting it has been. Lord Byron wrote in his journal:

> When one subtracts from life infancy (which is vegetation), sleep, eating, and swilling – buttoning and unbuttoning – how much remains of downright existence? The summer of a dormouse.[18]

Mind you, he did take three hours each day getting dressed. Ultimately, in the mystery of our birth, our living and our dying, we are alone, uniquely ourselves, a single and singular integrity. As we grow older we need to hold fast to that integrity and to those experiences which for us have proved true in a world of rapid and mind-blowing change, for we should not wish (again in Eliot's words) 'to have had the experience but missed the meaning'. To miss the meaning is to be blind to the fact that we are alone, yet not alone, for on our journey we carry others with us in our hearts and thoughts, as they carry us. Thomas Traherne writes that 'A private person is but half himself, and naturally multiplied in others.' And all the great Faiths in their different ways affirm that the whole point of our lives is to open ourselves to others in the give and take of love as the only way of expressing our humanity and thereby opening ourselves to God. This mutual exchange is the door to the final awareness of the unity of all things and all people in the dance of creation. There are a number of ways in which I may imagine the shape of my life, both its inner as well as its outer journey. I can see it simply as a *straight line* from birth to death, emerging from darkness and going back into darkness. Or I may picture it as a *circle*. There is the natural cycle of the seasons, echoing the rhythm of my life: the growth and vigour of spring; the richness and maturity of summer; the gradual diminishment of autumn, the time of harvest and the falling of the leaves; the bleak, but often beautiful landscape of winter, when the shape of trees becomes so much clearer. And the autumn and winter of our lives are the time when we begin to come full circle, when (in Eliot's words from 'Little Gidding')

> ... the end of all our exploring
> Will be to arrive where we started
> And know the place for the first time.[19]

But perhaps best of all, I can add the dimension of height (and by implication, depth) and see my life as a slowly ascending *spiral*. For a spiral suggests a life where each new circle – each new year or decade – still contains within it the make-up of the old, the feeling of familiarity, the octogenarian still aware of what it *felt* like to be the child, the lover, the parent he or she once was, and still displaying the same recognisable characteristics, but wiser now, shaped by life's knocks, able to say, 'I have been here before and learned a thing or two.' Looking back, we can begin to understand our own unique story and see that we have been moving in a spiral round a centre. At the centre of every circle there is a still point. For Christians that still point at the centre of our lives is the God whose creative spirit undergirds his whole creation, the God whose nature is 'a circle whose centre is everywhere and the circumstance nowhere'; and whose affirming love is made known in Jesus Christ.

This small poem by the American writer Raymond Carver, written not long before he died too young of cancer, is now much quoted:

> And did you get what you wanted from life, even so?
> I did.
> And what did you want?
> To know myself beloved, to feel myself
> beloved on the earth.[20]

The need to be affirmed, to feel ourselves of value, even beloved, is part of what it means to be human. There are few better nouns to describe the ministry of Jesus of Nazareth than 'affirmation'. Individual after individual crosses his path needing some kind of healing, and goes away affirmed, knowing that because they matter in his eyes, they matter equally to God. We each have our own stories and we each need at times to share our stories. All centre on the need to love and be loved, to be fulfilled in our search for what speaks to us of the good, the true and the lasting in the tangled yarn of our lives. And nowhere is this truer than when we reflect on our mortality, or when we come to die. In one sense it's true that, in the words of the funeral service, 'we brought nothing into this world and we can take nothing out', but that applies to the clutter of money and possessions and attachments; for in a deeper sense, what we take out is *not* nothing: it's a life given by God which (for the lucky ones) over the years has been shaped by our genes and desires and people and events, and then – if we so desire – offered back to God to be used, in ways known only to him, to his glory and the growth of his Kingdom. One of my predecessors at Westminster Abbey, Dean Eric Abbott, wrote:

> When we come to the end ... God will be able to take what we have done for him, whether implicitly or explicitly, and will gather it into his Kingdom, to be in that Kingdom that particular enrichment of the Kingdom's glory which our particular life has to contribute. *For there is something which only you can bring into the Kingdom.*[21] [My italics.]

'Men must endure their going hence,' says Edgar in *King Lear*; 'even as their coming hither: Ripeness is all.' In similar vein, immediately before the duel that will lead to his death, Hamlet says to Horatio: 'If it be now, 'tis not to come; if it be not to come, it will be now; if it be not now, yet it will come: the readiness is all.'[22] I come back to Helen Luke on *King Lear*, that seminal play about old age. The 80-year-old Lear, through his foolish need to know how much his three daughters love him, and his refusal to accept his increasing inability to exercise power, loses his kingdom and all but loses his mind: 'O! let me not be mad, not mad, sweet heaven; keep me in temper: I would not be mad.' But he comes through his suffering, finds again the faithful Cordelia, and in some of the loveliest and tenderest lines Shakespeare ever wrote expresses the essence of old age:

> Come, let's away to prison:
> We two alone will sing like birds i' the cage:
> When thou dost ask me blessing, I'll kneel down
> And ask of thee forgiveness: so we'll live,
> And pray, and sing, and tell old tales, and laugh
> At gilded butterflies, and hear poor rogues
> Talk of court news: and we'll talk with them too, –
> Who loses and who wins; who's in, who's out; –
> And take upon's the mystery of things
> As if we were God's spies; and we'll wear out,
> In a walled prison, packs and scores of great ones,
> That ebb and flow by th'moon.[23]

In her book, Helen Luke sees these 12 lines from the end of *Lear* as containing all the essential wisdom into which we may hope to grow in our declining years. 'Come, let's away to prison': not so much an actual prison as the seeming imprisonment of old age, with its failing powers and limitations, which we can either fight or learn to embrace, truly *growing* into the final flowering and meaning of our lives. 'We too alone will sing like birds i' the cage.' Cordelia is not simply Lear's youngest, most honest daughter: she is also a symbol of innocence. He has rejected her love for him, a love to which he now blessedly returns, able like a singing bird to sing out his love in response. So that 'When thou dost ask me blessing, I'll kneel down and ask of thee forgiveness.' Forgiveness – of ourselves, of each other, of the old by the young and the young by the old – is the only healing balm that brings peace of mind and true spiritual growth. 'So we'll live, And pray, and sing, and tell old tales, and laugh at gilded butterflies ...' Here are the proper occupations of old age: that giving attention which lies at the heart of prayer; feeding on good memories but also living for the moment that is now; and the laughter of pure delight at moments of gratuitous beauty. 'And hear poor rogues talk of court news; and we'll talk with them too, – who loses and who wins, who's in, who's out.' We need to retain a lively and curious interest in the world about us and its passing fashions. There follow two of the most wonderful lines Shakespeare ever wrote: 'And take upon's the mystery of things, As if we were God's spies.' A spy is one who seeks to penetrate into a hidden mystery, and God's spies are those who know intuitively that the whole world is his; that this is a sacramental creation, where (in the words of William Blake) 'everything that lives is holy'; that all is indeed mystery and that, if only we know how to look, everything we see is touched by wonder. So that, finally: 'We'll wear out, In a wall'd prison, packs and sects of great ones, that ebb and flow by th'moon.' We may be in the 'wall'd prison' of old age, but no longer at the beck and call of ambition, or the will to power, or the greed, or the need to control and manipulate, that sets the world's agenda, and so we can find a kind of liberation in small pleasures, in the telling of old tales, just in *being*, in the knowledge that the rocket, the terrorist and the bomb which dominate the nightly news can never in the end prevail over the gilded butterfly, or the 'unremembered acts of kindness and of love'.

The time will come when

> the grasshopper shall be a burden, and desire shall fail; because man goeth to his long home, and the mourners go about the streets: Or ever the silver cord be loosed, or the golden bowl be broken, or the pitcher be broken at the fountain, or the wheel broken at the cistern.
>
> Then shall the dust return to the earth as it was: and the spirit shall return unto God who gave it.[24]

If, as we grow old and desire with all our being truly to *grow* as we age, then we may indeed come to understand that 'the readiness is all'; and that 'all in the end is harvest'.[25]

The Questioning Country of Cancer

Certainly it is heaven upon earth, to have a ...
mind move in charity, rest in providence, and turn
upon the poles of truth.

Francis Bacon

What a minefield
Life is! One minute you're taking a stroll in the sun,
The next your legs and arms are all over the hedge,
There's no dignity in it.

Christopher Fry[1]

Laugh where we must, be candid where we can;
But vindicate the ways of God to man.

Alexander Pope[2]

... in sickness and in health ...

Book of Common Prayer

Shortly after I had written Parts I and II in my confident
retirement, the cancer struck.

Why did it happen? Cancer of the jaw is rare in non-
smokers or in people who don't drink to excess. Could it
have started 30 years ago when week after week, for seven
years, I attended three-hour-long, heads-of-department

meetings at the BBC in a deeply smoke-filled room? Or when ten years later, convalescing after M.E., I spent several days in Innsbruck when it was severely affected by radioactive dust from Chernobyl? Is it connected to the two malignant melanomas of ten years ago? Surely not. But whatever the reason, it announced itself in the summer of 2005.

For ten months I had suffered a recurrence of the M.E. that had put me out of action for a while in the 1980s: the familiar weakness, the muscular aches and pains, the evening nausea, the general diminishment; but it began to lift in June 2005. For months I had had a swelling under my tongue, which V., my dentist, didn't think would clear up until the M.E. had burned itself out. X-rays in April showed nothing sinister. But it grew worse, and an X-ray in June showed an ominous change. She at once referred me to a consultant, Ian Downie, at the Salisbury Hospital Oral Clinic. I warmed to him at once. 'I will tell you everything you ask me,' he said. 'If there's something I don't know, I'll say so.' In situations like this, there are things you *need* to know and things you don't *want* to know, but it's better that you should. Luckily, Southampton Hospital is the regional centre in the south-west for the treatment of head and neck cancer, and Salisbury Hospital is linked to it. A biopsy was taken from under my tongue and I was asked to return on 4th July. It was an anxious week, in which everything seemed to be on 'pause'. What follows is as honest as I can make it.

4th July
Appointed morning Psalm, 9: 'I will give thanks to you, Lord, with my whole heart; I will tell of all your marvellous works ...' Can't say it (yet) with any great conviction. I.D. confirms that the biopsy shows cancer. Sense of shock, though half-expected. He is uncertain if it has gone into the bone and/or to left or right lymph nodes. Spells out with infinite care what he plans to do. We have the option of Salisbury or Southampton for the long, intricate operation.

At the latter he would be part of the team; if here, he would be the chief surgeon. Come home very subdued. Phone family.

5th July

Morning Psalm, 56: 'Whenever I am afraid, I will put my trust in you ... for what can flesh do to me?' Try to relay it from head to heart. To hospital for chest X-ray, CT scan of head and shoulders, blood tests. Graham, our GP, calls in and spells out some further details. Calmer, though a bit panicky. Type out, covering all possibilities, details of choice of funeral service. Should have done it years ago. Remember John Robinson, godfather to our daughter Sarah, preaching in Trinity Chapel when diagnosed with inoperable cancer on the question of whether 'God is in the cancer'. Will brood on this and hopefully write about it. Can I learn to consider cancer as a gift? How can it be redeemed, good brought out of it? Shaky and cold tonight. At dusk the beautiful swifts slice through the sky and a songthrush fills the air with its haunting music.

6th July

Wake at 3 a.m. (the nadir of the night). Splitting headache. The reality hits you afresh each day on waking. Morning Psalm, 57: 'Be merciful to me, O God, be merciful, for I have taken refuge in you; in the shadow of your wings will I take refuge until this time of trouble has gone by.' A. and I walk by River Avon: wonderful scent of wild roses. Moments of panic and mild nausea. 'Thou wilt keep him in perfect peace, whose mind is stayed on thee.' Yes: but at times the mind refuses to be stayed. The thrush in fine voice again at dusk.

7th July

These days of waiting are testing. No decisions about when and where the operation will be for another few days. Phone calls to friends take their toll: such varied reactions. Mark

Bonney comes. Long talk, prays and blesses me. Importance of touch. Christina Shewell comes from Bristol with gifts of heliotrope and tayberries. A kind of mild nausea persists: occasionally the heart lurches as the imagination unhelpfully explores the unpredictable. Each day, like Pope's wounded snake, 'drags its slow length along'. As a priest, I'm all too familiar with hospitals, yet only briefly until now as a patient. Deep down, I want to see this time as a gift to be used fruitfully: on the surface, head doesn't yet match heart. Ashamed to be self-obsessed on a terrible day of bombs on London Underground and a bus, with many deaths and casualties. In the garden, the roses are in full bloom, the bees bothering the lavender. Elsewhere, the mindless destruction.

8th July

Morning Psalm, 59: 'You have become my stronghold, a refuge in the day of my trouble. To you, O my Strength, will I sing; for you, O God, are my stronghold and my merciful God.' To Bake Farm to pick raspberries. It's hard, this period of waiting, for when the unpredictable happens in a reasonably settled life, there's no time to prepare. But now there is: images of surgery, discomfort, helplessness, lodge in the mind. Mouth very sore, a nagging reminder of the shock in store for it. Am fearful, not of dying – I.D. has told my GP he thinks it 'curable' – but of coping. Must see it as a way of transmuting an unwelcome invasion into something to be used creatively. Tonight the swifts are noisier than ever, their flight the epitome of grace.

9th July

Wake early: my brain worries away at imagining my post-operative state. 'Be still, my soul' – but the mind has a life of its own. I know both too much and not enough. The Psalms – 63 this morning – never cease to come up trumps: 'My soul is content ... when I remember you upon my bed, and meditate upon you in the night watches. For you have been my helper, and under the shadow of your wings I will rejoice.' If only . . . Feel low all day. Yet calmness on my part will best help those closest to me. This is a test of all that my life has tried to bear witness to, all those years of counselling and preaching and seeking to live out that *cantus firmus* which I claim to be central and authentic. My enduring melody. The time for my words to become flesh. Visit the sculpture garden at nearby Roche Court: a fine new slate feature by Richard Long. Feel in limbo. A feverish night sees the start of a painful bladder infection.

10th July

Spend most of day in bed. Duty doctor comes: prescribes antibiotics. The hottest day of the summer: swifts flying non-stop outside the window the sole refreshment.

11th July

Still feverish. Up hourly in night. Could do without this. Time creeps. 'Lead me from despair to hope, from fear to trust.'

12th July

Morning Psalm, 62: 'For God alone my soul in silence waits; truly, my hope is in him. He alone is my rock and my salvation, my stronghold, so that I shall not be shaken.' Sarah joins us for visit to cancer unit in Southampton. An hour in humid, crowded waiting-room. Then an hour of impeccable attention from consultant and registrar. They think it's a primary cancer which may have begun to spread into the bone. During the surgery they plan to replace part of the lower jaw with flesh, nerves and artery from the inner wrist; they will also remove a selection of lymph nodes from ear to ear. If they show signs of cancer six weeks of radiotherapy follow. 'Have I an option?' 'Yes, a combination of radio- and chemotherapy.' No, thanks. Cancer team very impressive. Decide to opt for the operation at Salisbury (smaller, near home) and, as main surgeon, I.D. who impresses us more and more. Feeling of relief when more details known and decision made. '... So that I shall not be shaken.' But we can't fail to be.

13th July
Morning Psalm, 63: 'My soul clings to you; your right hand holds me fast.' Letter from Mother Mary John of West Malling Benedictine community. Promises the prayers of the community, as have the other two communities I know best: Burford and Tymawr. Good to be undergirded with the prayers of the professionally religious. They know how to do it. Very hot still, but feel more human. Diana Roberts comes with raspberries. 'What is real piety?' asks Sydney Smith in a letter to Mrs Baring in 1834. 'What is true attachment to the Church? How are these fine feelings best evinced? The answer is plain: by sending strawberries to a clergyman.'[3] But raspberries will do. At lunchtime I.D. phones: important to proceed as soon as possible, hopefully in two days' time, which means going into hospital tomorrow. Will phone back. 'Your right hand holds me fast' battles with moments of panic. Prepare some CDs to take in and write and file hasty but heartfelt letters to A., Mark and Sarah, 'just in case'. But it is a false alarm. They cannot collect team together so soon. Confirms Friday week – Feast of St Mary Magdalen, first witness to the resurrection. A good omen? Oppressive night. Christopher, brother of my valued friend of 20 years, Cicely Saunders, phones to say she is unlikely to last the night. I spoke to her five days ago, the last day when she was fully conscious, and we said our goodbyes.

14th July
Telephone some close friends: one asks the length of the operation. 'I've been told 12 hours at least.' His response ('Jeeper's creepers!') and that of the second an hour later ('Good God!') aren't exactly consoling. Drive to Roche Court and spend time in the flower-filled walled garden. Reluctantly cancel tickets for *Henry IV* at the National Theatre.

Reflecting on God (1)

'The questioning country of cancer' brings with it the renewed sense that this is a test. A test of what A. and I most deeply believe about the undergirding presence of God; of our own inner resources; of how something so major is to be accepted and integrated into the continuing story of our lives. It needs to be made to fit, a natural part of the overall journey. Having never believed in a God who could prevent cancer, or who, like some temperamental Greek god, flings thunderbolts around, I don't ask, 'Why me?' Our freedom – and that of the whole natural order with its established laws which yet allow an element of chance, a certain randomness and choice, including the freedom to go wrong – prevents it. No doubt God could have created a perfect world, free of pain and sickness, in which its creatures were programmed to lead model lives and sing his praises through all eternity. But that perfect creation would be God's mirror, not his companion, a perversion of the give-and-take of love. Love is only love when it is willingly and freely given. This is not the time to philosophise or rehearse theological defences of an often perplexing world. It's the time to find God in the love and prayerful concern of family and friends, in the skill of microsurgery and the care of doctors and nurses in what is patently an outstanding team. I glimpse him when I really focus on certain affirming phrases, in the calmness that ensues, and in the sense of being upheld and stilled instead of my mind racing round like a hamster in a wheel.

This is *my* illness, *my* cancer, and the form it takes is peculiar to me. The medical team seem to recognise this, sensing what and how much to say. My reactions to it – a dislike of blood and scalpels – stem from childhood experiences, starting with having my tonsils out, in Abdication Year, aged seven, very messily with gas, strapped down on the kitchen table. My anxieties are a mixture of good and bad: good ones like a concern for A. and the family, the stress they will be under, the worry of friends. Seemingly trivial ones like the length of the anaesthetic, the likely nausea, the fear of feverish dreams and nightmares. Will the catheter stay in place? Will my bowels work? Will I be able to speak properly again? For how long will I feel weak as a kitten? Will I lose my sense of taste and smell? *All* my teeth? And what about pain control? Some of this you can ask the doctors (though not always welcoming the answers); some you can't if you want to retain a scrap of dignity. Like all of us, I'm a double person: one part is immature and panicky, the other mature and in control. I don't want to lose my awareness of how lucky we are to live in the developed world, or my gratitude that so many friends and communities in such scattered places are praying for me. I see them as candles burning in the dark. The words near the end of *King Lear* keep coming to mind: 'I have a journey, sir, shortly to go; my master calls me, I must not say no.' And Hamlet's 'The readiness is all.' (Only later shall we know if it has crept further in its destructive course, which will mean the tedious daily sessions of radiotherapy.) Meanwhile I believe this cancer will be cured. I go into the coming weeks with that confidence. At least, I do while it's still a long, difficult week away.

How self-centred all this is! Inevitable, I guess. Not helped by so many phone calls, and the constant repetition of the facts. One of the verses from today's set Psalm (116) is: 'Turn again to your rest, O my soul, for the Lord has treated you well.' How many thousand times have I used the words before sleep, 'Father, into your hands I commend my spirit' with a comfortable sense of untroubled security: now I must try to do so with open hands and a calm mind.

15th July
To the Oral Clinic at Salisbury Hospital to see I.D., two colleagues and a nurse. He goes through all that he plans to do in minute detail, much of it a necessary repeat of Southampton, for the brain only remembers selectively in such circumstances. He listens attentively to every question. Half the skill in medical practice lies in the gift of

51

communication. A surgeon's skill is so like an artist's: precise, meticulous, giving rapt attention. It must be strange to invade so aggressively and intimately the body of a near-stranger. The current heatwave (non-air-conditioned hospital) doesn't help. Return at 2 for blood tests, ECG tests and ultrasound. Extraordinary to watch the blood surging through your veins on a computer screen.

Tiring day. Every day over 700 people in this country are told they have cancer, and for some it is terminal. With the diagnosis of a life-threatening illness you enter into a different world and it quickly takes you over. At least after this, I can say what only living through one of the major life experiences can entitle you to say: 'I have been there and I *know*.' Though not, hopefully, the terminal bit: that calls for a different kind of courage.

The thrush, along with the blackbirds, has stopped singing (and won't sing again for seven months). Our single old apple tree, which has given me such delight during the past somewhat sedentary year as a staging-post for greenfinch and siskin, chaffinch and goldfinch, and our faithful pair of collared doves (six meals a day, clownishly balanced side-by-side on the small feeder), is slowly dying.

16th July

Our children and grandchildren come. Until you're old you can't imagine how strange it is to realise that their very existence turns on something as trivial as a chance meeting 40 years ago. Each day friends ring: others, more helpfully, write. Some, even more helpfully, add: 'Don't reply.' The most succinct card, from a Roman Catholic friend, reads: 'My God, what a bugger!' Spot on. Calmer now, but occasional moments of panic which, just by snapping its fingers, can at once obliterate the solid ground of trust and confidence I strive for. I must remain *curious*, curious to learn more of the mystery of the body, and of my belief in my relationship with the love which lies at the very heart of my life, to the source of which I give the name 'God'.

17th July

To the cathedral Eucharist. The set Psalm is 139:1–11. The perfect words to accompany me this week:

> If I climb up to heaven, you are there; if I make the grave my bed, you are there also ... even there your hand will lead me and your right hand hold me fast. If I say, 'Surely the darkness will cover me, and the light around me turn to night', darkness is not dark to you; the night is as bright as the day; darkness and light to you are both alike.

My disobedient mind keeps returning to the night before the op., and A. leaving, and the unpredictable days in intensive care. I'm like a sparrow perched on a branch keeping a wary eye open for the circling hawk, panic, which may swoop down at the least expected moment and chill the blood. Very hot tonight. Lying in bed, watch the clouds drifting across the three-quarter moon. But they hold no promise of refreshing rain.

18th July

Psalm 102:4–12: wonderfully evocative set of metaphors describing a sense of distress:

> My days are consumed in smoke ... My heart is smitten down and withered like grass, so that I forget to eat my bread ... My bones cleave fast to my skin. I am become like a vulture in the wilderness, like an owl that haunts the ruins ... I am become like a sparrow solitary upon the housetop ... I have eaten ashes for bread and mingled my drink with weeping ... My days fade away like shadow and I am withered like grass.

Disturbing letter in the *Independent* from nurse in Poole. Says local hospital has no air-conditioning, ward temperatures are 39 degrees, patients lying in pools of sweat. A. as caring as ever, but looks so stressed and can think of little else. Glad that this is happening to me, not her. An anonymous twelfth-century Irish hermit wrote this on the cost of watching one you love suffer: 'Ah, sore was the suffering borne by the body of Mary's son, but sorer still to him was the grief which for his sake came upon his mother.'

Ted Heath has died. Remember when he came to supper in Cambridge in the 1980s before speaking brilliantly on the Brandt Report in Great St Mary's, and our dog had eaten all the steak and kidney from the kitchen table an hour earlier. He had to put up with pasta. Not our finest hour, and – as he made all too clear – not his, but funny in retrospect. Hope he is less grumpy, and finds consoling music, in heaven.

Sixty cards and letters already, a great help. My 'mantras' in hospital won't be the Jesus Prayer with its constant emphasis on our sinfulness, but (i) the verse from 'St Patrick's Breastplate':

> Christ be with me, Christ within me,
> Christ behind me, Christ before me,
> Christ beside me, Christ to win me,
> Christ to comfort and restore me.
>
> Christ beneath me, Christ above me,
> Christ in quiet, Christ in danger,
> Christ in hearts of all who love me,
> Christ in mouth of friend and stranger.

(ii) The words of Boethius that I had painted round the walls of the Deanery 'Abbots' Pew' chapel at Westminster:

> To see thee is the end and the beginning,
> Thou carriest me and thou goest before;
> Thou art the journey and the journey's end.

(iii) St Paul's words to the young church at Philippi: 'I can do all things through Christ who strengthens me'; and
(iv) Julian of Norwich's phrase, that we are 'enfolded in God', enfolded in love. Only that which has proved authentic in the past will serve.

John and Jill Baker come, armed with white orchid. He was Tutor at Cuddesdon 50 years ago, and a wonderful friend ever since. He encourages me to write and tell it 'as it is'.

19th July

Set Psalm, 119. In Hugh's 'christianised' version[4] verse 109 reads: 'I live each day on the edge of darkness, But I know you will hold me in your mercy.' Appropriate collect for this week (Trinity 8) asking God to so 'direct our hearts and bodies in the ways of your laws and the works of your commandments, that through your most mighty protection … we may be preserved in body and soul'.

Reflecting on prayer (1)

During this past year of M.E. and now the cancer diagnosis, I've tried (not always very successfully) to focus on the grace of God and on gratitude. In past years I've taken so much for granted. Twenty more letters and cards this morning, making me aware of much supportive prayer. Can it possibly affect the outcome? The laws of nature are mercifully constant and dependable; without radical treatment the cancer will run its deadly course unchecked and (the jaw getting more tender daily) I long to be shot of the diseased part. Yet if (as I believe in my reflective moments) it is 'in God that we (*all*) live and move and have our being', I see prayer as being the expression of that truth, the conscious uniting with that deep centre of life and healing of me and those whom I love and who love me, together with the surgeons, doctors, nurses, who will treat me. Putting my human vulnerability and their skills into a broader context in which the life-giving forces are enabled to work most effectively. I believe that behind all healing is our ability to tap into the creative source of life itself who once, in Jesus, took on that vulnerability. In the ever-present image of that crucified man we have the ultimate mystery of how human suffering reveals God's compassion, the seeming paradox of the Creator shown in a moment of time to be as vulnerable as any of his defenceless creatures.

What I face is as nothing compared with the daily anguish of millions, the impossible-to-visualise suffering of the AIDS-stricken continent of Africa, the endless slaughter in Iraq, the unheard cries of the tortured and oppressed. In comparison, I am shamefully privileged to live in comfort, the best medical skill to hand (and free), surrounded by loving support. Remembering this puts the coming weeks and months into proportion. Yet human nature 'cannot bear very much reality', and when illness knocks you flat you become a citizen of the shrunken, private world of the sick, your self-concern for yourself and those you love putting all else temporarily on hold. There's nothing shameful about being obsessively aware for a while of your own mortality, especially if that brings with it a desire to meet the test as creatively as you can.

Bishop Peter comes. A good listener. Tells me that his daughter, a dentist, was called in to take part in my exact operation. She was so moved and inspired by the surgeon's skill that she is now training to be a doctor. He reflects on how fortuitous are the circumstances that have brought me, from the moment of my birth, and the members of my surgical team, from the moment of each of theirs, together in this place for this long day of surgery. Seen in worldly terms, it is pure chance; but perhaps, in the long unfolding providence of God, it is part of the design for my journey, and theirs. Part of the invisible side of the tapestry, of which we can now only see knots and loose ends. Well, maybe: it's a comforting thought. But God's providential love implies our absolute freedom, and it could easily have been otherwise: the same me, but in a different setting and with a different cast.

Looking after the family's labrador, Camas, for six weeks. Walk by the river, where she swims and swims. Fields already brown with harvest. Reed bunting and wrens flit through the rushes; swallows skim the surface.

20th July

Last day at home. This morning's Psalm, 119:133–134: H.'s 'christianised' version helpful:

> Keep my footsteps in the way that leads to life,
> And guard me from the powers of darkness.
> Rescue me from the fears that oppress me,
> So I may put my trust in your providence.

Drive to New Forest. Walk near Fritham Lake. Stonechats; many foals; the early heather in flower in small patches. Feel calm most of the time, though the unruly mind nags away at the thought of the coming days like the tongue at a jarring tooth. And the hawk panic still waits to pounce like the buzzards quartering this patch of forest. Call in at the tiny, unspoilt King's Arms for a pint of Ringwood Best, in case I lose my taste. On the answerphone a timely, affirming message from Fr Gerry Hughes, whose books have meant so much to me, saying that he read, and was encouraged by, mine when he was convalescing from a serious operation last year.

Read again some of Rilke's *Book of Hours, Love Poems to God*, which are pervaded by his sense of the divine presence, the accompanying Other, holding and supporting him:

> Don't you sense me, ready to break
> into being at your touch?[5]

He writes of pain as 'the terrible darkness that makes me small' and out of his pain addresses God:

> If it's you, though –
> press down hard on me, break in
> that I may know the weight of your hand,
> and you, the fulness of my cry.[6]

And he is good on the 'holy in the ordinary', believing we are able to redeem the world bit by bit through an act of *transforming attention*, that to name each tiny part of it is an act of love:

> I know that nothing has ever been real
> Without my beholding it.
> All becoming has needed me.
> My looking ripens things
> And they come toward me, to meet and be met.[7]

Which must include the cancer cells that work even now like a mole in the dark of my flesh. Which is why I seek to give every bit of this new experience my proper attention: to name it, and in so doing to name the God who is with me in it, not least in those who are giving both A. and me their attention and holding us in their love.

An almost full moon tonight. Wake at 2 with it shining full on our bed.

21st July

As I say my form of morning prayer a neighbour's dog is howling, and I think: 'Yes, a bit of me is howling too, but deeper there is a steady sense of being held and encouraged by many expressions of loving support.' (The root of 'encouragement' is the French *coeur*: literally to put 'heart' into someone, and it does.) Set Gospel reading, Luke 13:1–10 (the falling tower of Siloam and the barren fig-tree), pretty useless. But the collect for tomorrow, Mary Magdalen's Day, is good:

> Almighty God, whose Son restored Mary Magdalen to health of mind and body and called her to be a witness to his resurrection: forgive our sins and heal us by your grace, that we may serve you in the power of his risen life ...

Mark B. comes at 11 to anoint us and give us Communion. The ministry of touch goes very deep when you're sick. Our own Mark has given me a card to show to importunate visitors in the early days: 'I am very tired. Thank you for your visit.' Due at the hospital at 2 p.m. Phone the ward at 1:

'Sorry, but we're still trying to find you a bed.'

'Is there any doubt?'

'I hope not: I'll phone you back.'

But they don't for another two hours. Then: 'Is that Revd Payne?' Doesn't boost my confidence. There is a bed, but not until 4. 'Come at 3.30.' So it's all stations go. On arrival we're asked to sit in a small, hot waiting-room for an hour with an anxious, depressed family. Made to feel unwelcome. Finally given a bed in mixed eight-bed ward. See anaesthetist, plastic surgeon, I.D. He explains that my operation was only first pioneered 20 years ago, warns that it has a five per cent failure rate, and they will only know if the arteries and nerves have taken after two or three days. Also warns me that there still might be no bed in Intensive Care Unit. If none become free, he will do a less radical operation, bringing down two slices of cheek into the lower mouth, and the time in the ICU won't be necessary. Nothing is ever simple. L., the Oral Clinic sister, also warns me that after such a long anaesthetic I may be depressed, irritable and will for many weeks be extremely weak. A challenge to prove them wrong, at least about the first two. Sarah arrives, and she and A. leave at 8.

Within two minutes Bishop P. arrives, and is quietly affirming. Two women opposite. Woman number one eyes me with deep suspicion: the combination of a man visiting me out of hours wearing a purple stock plus me writing my journal ('Is he writing about me?' Well, yes, as it happens) is a bit much for her. Woman number two sits weeping gently, clutching her teddy bear. A nurse comforts her. Later, woman number one tries to speak to her but is sharply reprimanded: 'Go away! Can't you see I'm reading my book?' She is absorbed in a catalogue of garden plants.

Read a few of William Maxwell's short stories without taking in a word; then the night office, Compline. Psalm 91 helpful:

> He who dwells in the shelter of the Most High,
> abides under the shadow of the Almighty ...
> You shall not be afraid of any terror by night,

nor of the arrow that flies by day;
Of the plague that stalks in the darkness,
nor of the sickness that lays waste at midday.

Repeat, with a newly realised fervour: 'I can do all things' – endure all things – 'through Christ who strengthens me.' Too old for teddy bears.

22nd July

Sleep for an hour about midnight. Ward pretty quiet. Woman number two laughs loudly in her sleep. Awake from 1–4 a.m., then remember ear-plugs and sleep until woken at 6. Sense of unreality during the small hours of the night: will it really be 'me' on that table in the morning with comparative strangers slicing me up? Couldn't I just slip quietly home? Woman number two now panicky and weeping: they are so good and patient with her. Long to comfort A. at home, who won't have slept much. Say collect for Eastertide to celebrate Mary Magdalen, Psalm 139:1–5 , and the words from the Song of Songs:

Set me as a seal upon your heart,
as a seal upon your arm;
For love is strong as death,
passion fierce as the grave ...
Many waters cannot quench love,
neither can the floods drown it.

At this exact moment, in the lovely Trinity chapel in the cathedral, many friends will be starting morning prayer and the Eucharist, Mark B. celebrating, and I am being remembered. Never have the words 'pray, love, remember' (prayer, *agape*, and the Eucharist) as the central demands of the Christian life been more meaningful. And then it begins to fall apart. They like you now to *walk* to the Anaesthetics Room, but suddenly I am overwhelmed by dizziness and nausea, and go by the less dignified horizontal route. The op. was due to start at 8; it's now 8.45 ...

A., waiting with Sarah and Mark, got her phone call from I.D. to say that I was back from theatre at 9.45 that evening. Thank God for modern anaesthetics and morphine, but you pay a price in the wild, hallucinatory days and nights that follow while it is working its way out of your system. What follows is the family's account of the next few days; but first, Ian Downie's account, in medical terms, of what was done.

Procedures

Neck dissection: infiltration with 2x20 mls 1% Lignocaine with 1:200,000 Adrenaline. Upper flap raised. A highly suspicious node in the left submandibular (1) region. Mandibular (2) branch of facial nerve clearly identified. Lower border of mandible (3) exposed. Excision of tumour. Soft tissue dissection with Colorado (4). Mandibular rim resection lower right 4 to lower 3 left 3. Frozen sections taken from 1) anterior 2) right posterior margin, 3) left posterior margin and 4) deep margin. All were clear. Bony resection between mental foramen (5) and to include all the roots of the anterior teeth. Cuts were made with bur (6) and completed with Epkar osteotome (7). Sublingual (8) glands were excised and ducts ligated (9) with 3/0 Vicryl. A left supraomohyoid (10) dissection completed. Preservation of nerves X, XI and XII. Submandibular gland removed. Lingual gland nerve identified and preserved. Right submandibular triangle cleared. Floor of mouth reconstructed with an ALT flap done by Mr Downie and Miss McGuinness. Inset with 4/0 Vicryl rapide (11).

Free left anterplateral (12) thigh flap to mouth: 3x5 cm ALT flap (13) from left thigh raised on two perforators (14). Donor site closed directly with 3/0 Vicryl and 3/0 Monocryl with 18 gauge. Flap inset to mouth with 4/0 Vicryl rapide (15).

Micro: LCFA (16) to suprathyroid (17) artery (left) end-to-end (9/0 Ethylon). LCFV (18) to IJV (19) end-to-side (9/0 Ethylon). LCFV (20) to IJV branch end-to-end (9/0 Ethylon).

Layman's key: *(1) Of the lower jaw. (2) Of the lower jaw. (3) Lower jaw. (4) A specific type of diathermy (cutting with a very hot needle). (5) Small hole in the lower jaw which the nerve supplying sensation to the lip exits. (6) Drill bit. (7) Eponymous chisel. (8) Under the tongue. (9) Tied up. (10) Describes the area above the omohyoid muscle running from low down in the neck to a bone in the midline just below the lower jaw. (11) A resorbing stitch. (12) Tissue from the front/outer part of the thigh. (13) Ditto. (14) Perforators: small blood vessels supplying an area of bone. (14–15) This refers to: (i) the 'donor' site on the thigh from which the graft was harvested was closed with a single resorbable stitch under the skin; and (ii) the graft was stitched into the mouth with multiple individual resorbable stitches. (16–20) Abbreviations for arteries and veins in the leg and neck.*

(All that took 12 hours. The first of the post-operative notes read: 'Flap observations every 15 minutes for first 24 hours, then 30 mins for second 24 hours.' Within a short time there were problems developing: a haemotoma which could have become a blood clot proved disastrous, and I was back in theatre for another couple of hours later that night. It happened again in the morning, and I returned to theatre for a further hour. Luckily I knew nothing.)

Alison writes

When we first heard Michael's diagnosis, almost my first thought is that I need my mother, who died in February, as she would make it all better. I then realised it was a great relief not to have to tell her about M.'s illness, and that we were facing this together, although he would go through it alone. And it does feel as if we are leaving him all alone in a crowded ward when Sarah and I say goodbye to him on Thursday evening, still not sure whether the planned surgery will go ahead at 8 a.m. the next day because of constant uncertainty over the availability of an Intensive Care Unit bed.

And so we get up on Friday morning following a very long night to a very long day; only Sarah's dog is unaware of our fears and greets us in the kitchen as cheerfully as ever. I am so grateful that Sarah is with me and that Mark arrives about midday. We lunch together at The Yew Tree in Odstock, in fact a short distance down the road from the hospital where M.'s operation is taking place. We eat clutching our mobiles, feeling isolated in the crowded pub amongst people who have no inkling of what is happening in our family. I find it almost unbearable to imagine what is being done to M. throughout the day – and yet I want to know. The day goes on, followed by a lengthy evening interspersed by friends telephoning, each of which we hope will be I.D. And finally at 21.42 he calls, explains that there was a delay in getting started this morning and that the op. has gone well and that he will see M. in the morning.

Following a wakeful night, Sarah phones the ICU and speaks to J., M's nurse, who explains that he was taken back to theatre during the early hours because of a bleed, but is now back. At 8.45 Sarah, Mark and I go to the hospital and find he is back in theatre again, so we go home for an anxious breakfast. We return at 10.30 and wait in the visitors' room outside the ward. At 11.30 I.D. arrives having seen M. and explains what has happened, which we find reassuring; and then at 11.45 we all go in to see M., with tubes, drains, machines that click and bleep, and with a very swollen face. Although he is sedated and seemingly unaware, he is also in a strange way present, and there we sit with him holding his hands, and feel as if we have stepped off the real world into this enclosed bubble of intensive care which is to be his home for a while. The staff make us welcome, so we do not feel in the way as they constantly monitor his progress while we sit round the bed. It is helpful when the nurse caring for him explains to us, and also to M. when he is conscious and even before this, what she is going to do for him and why. This underlines how vital communication is: what is accepted as routine and obvious in the medical world needs spelling out for us in layman's language so that we can be involved and aware. And almost before he is fully conscious M. is struggling to communicate by writing largely illegible messages on a pad.

Throughout this whole experience so far, the sharing of information (encouraging or not) has made it possible to bear, with M., what has happened and what may lie ahead. Also, of course, the presence and imaginative support for us both of Sarah and Mark.

Sarah writes

When I look back now at those four days when Dad was being operated upon and recovering in Intensive Care, I am left with a series of images. The first is of catching Dad's eye as Mum and I left him in the hospital ward, knowing that the next time we saw him, he would have come through an immensely long and complex operation. As a nurse I had some concept of what would be involved; as a daughter this was unknown territory.

The second memory is of a long night and an even longer day spent with Mum and Mark. We were all very anxious and we talked easily and gained strength from being together.

Walking into the Intensive Care Unit the next day, we found Dad very swollen and deeply sedated. Although he did not respond to us, sitting with him and being able to hold his hand was so much easier than the endless hours of waiting and ima-gining. One of the most powerful memories is of the care given by the nurses in Intensive Care. All were good but some were out-standing. The ability to know a person who you have only just met and never had a conversation with requires intuition of the highest order. The nurse who had understood Dad's sense of humour over the issue of being too hot in the night, by coming to an agreement with him when he pulled his blanket down each time her back was turned, that he might keep it down so long as he pulled it up as soon as either of them spotted a doctor on the ward, showed a level of understanding and empathy which brought us huge comfort and laughter.

Dad had planned for almost every eventuality, including establishing a code for hand squeezes. One squeeze for 'yes', two for 'no' and three for 'I love you'. Not only did we need to tell him we loved him during those first anxious days, but it also became an important bond between Anna and me. We had delayed leaving for an extended holiday in Europe, and set out four days after the operation, and as we walked through the towns of Eastern Europe during Dad's recovery, we would squeeze each

64

other's hands in multiples of three and know we were thinking of him.

By the time Anna and Adam visited on the Sunday, Dad was more responsive and he put a huge effort into reacting to them. We were going away the next day and he made sure that he wished them a good holiday and soon established a sign for swimming, a passion he shares with Anna. With huge insight, the children insisted that we took with us a photograph of Grandpa before his operation so that we would remember how he really looked.

Saying goodbye and leaving Dad in Intensive Care, and Mum with him, was one of the hardest things I have ever done. The moment, over a fortnight later, when my mobile rang on a very crowded tram in Krakow, with Dad's voice at the other end to say he was home, prompted almost as many tears – not to mention a few slightly bemused Polish commuters!

Mark writes

Like Humpty Dumpty set upon by a gang with baseball bats would be a better description than your consultant's warning that you are 'quite swollen'.

It's strange, this first meeting with you. Strange that you are sleeping, not screaming – given the ordeal – and incredible that surgery of such complexity and precision should create so much swelling and distortion. And yet it is still very much you that remains, resting underneath this cartoon version.

It's also strange for me to see you sleeping. I know you very well yet I am still surprised by this because it's unfamiliar. It's also strange, as with the operation itself, that the one person who has been at the centre of the anxiety is now oblivious to its outcome.

You will be resurfacing in fits and starts, trying to piece it all together, rather than hearing it directly from your consultant, as we do. And when you do, your first priority is to let us know how you are. Indeed, throughout the following days, we become deci-pherers of hand squeezes, letters spelt in the air and scribbled notes – for all of which you develop proficiency quickly –

reminding me of how crucial communication is for you, and the cruelty of this particular cancer.

While thankful to see you in one intricately sewn-together piece, I am then keen to get out before I pass out.

Mum kisses you and Sarah holds your hand. I feel sick, so I follow the tubes and colours pulsing on the monitors above your bed and also the movement of staff for any clues of panic or disaster. It's only on a second or third visit to ICU that I realise that it is not an emergency room as seen on TV and that patients are more likely to slip into a critical condition rather than be the centre of rapid rewiring and resuscitation by a team of fast-moving medics, as I'd first imagined.

You don't slip away and when you are out of ICU and on the ward, Mum comments on the fact that the whole experience has been rather like having a baby. You can only prepare to a certain point and then everything else is left to unknown outcomes and probably a certain degree of luck.

In these first few days, visiting you is challenging because you seem vulnerable and I don't really know what to do or say. It becomes more difficult when you are distressed, like when you feel as though you are suffocating, or when a brilliant nurse who you have built up a particular rapport with on one day is not looking after you the next.

These first few days in hospital are particularly memorable in what becomes a long haul. Writing this many months later, it seems that you have been particularly unlucky since the operation in your struggle to control the pain. It has been relentless. For someone who loves you, that's a hard thing to write about. I do know that you have written about it and for you it's a crucial part of the process. I guess that this may be one way for you to confront and perhaps transform it, not least through the way that your words will help to give some comfort to other readers. So I am delighted that you have allowed me a chance to contribute, as it is to you as a writer and not as a sufferer that I am sending these words.

Adam writes

The day on which we were due to leave the country (on a rear-ranged flight – one of the many results of Grandpa's illness), we went to visit him in Intensive Care. Dad was already in France and Mum had been in Salisbury for a few days, so Anna and I were driven down by our friend Tim with his obscure music collection.

On arrival at the hospital there was a definite air of anxiety, the hospital itself being extremely quiet this Sunday morning. Anna and I entered Intensive Care with Mum, having completed the necessary hand sterilisation, and saw Grandpa lying in a bed on the other side of a small room.

Physically he bore little resemblance to the Grandpa we knew and loved, but after a few seconds it became clear that it was just the superficial details that had changed. He insisted, in very 'Grandpa style', on writing almost unintelligible messages on a pad of paper as well as making one-armed swimming signs. Behind the swollen face and immobility lay, very definitely, our Grandpa. Of course, saying goodbye wasn't easy and it changed the nature of our holiday but, to use an overused cliché, we all knew that there was light at the end of the tunnel. The wonder of mobile technology and the knowledge that Grandpa would recover made the departure that bit easier.

*

Having attended the funeral of my dad's dad (who died of cancer while we were on holiday in Scotland) earlier this week, I have reflected on the nature of the last 12 months. Seeing both, see-mingly healthy, grandpas struck down by what is fundamentally the same disease, yet knowing that one will live and the other will die, has been surreal and an emotional roller-coaster.

Anna writes

When I think of what it was like seeing Grandpa in Intensive Care, the first thing I think of is him signing to me that he wanted me to do lots of swimming on the holiday on which we were about to go. Although it took a while to understand what he was signing, when you did, it was surprising how he signed just like Grandpa would talk, although he was very swollen and didn't look very much like himself.

On the way to the hospital I was nervous but when we got there that little bit of communication between me and Grandpa made it much easier. We were going away for the summer so it was hard to leave Grandpa, but afterwards I felt very glad that I went to see him.

23rd July

This day passed me by. I spent the next four days in Intensive Care. At first dreams and reality were interchangeable. I was aware of members of the family coming two by two, but could only grunt or write illegibly on a pad. The morphine continued to be pumped in and the hallucinations began: solid window frames turned liquid; the ceiling dissolved into a series of white sails. The clock on the far wall bent itself into strange, Daliesque shapes, and at night it kept on disintegrating, bits flying round the room. I heard voices just out of my area of vision calling me by name. These were no dreams, and therefore all the more discomfiting. On the third morning curtains were hurriedly drawn round the next bed. I heard, unmistakably, Alison in the bed talking to the nurse. She had had an accident on the way to see me and was seriously injured. 'What shall I do? My husband's in hospital; I'm looking after the family dog; our children have gone on holiday.'

I grew more and more anxious, and when the sister appeared, I beckoned her over. 'Where's my wife?'

'I hope she's in bed asleep: it's 6.45 in the morning.'

'Then who's in the next bed?'

'No one you know.'

That evening the sister produced a single get-well card sent to the hospital rather than home and hung it centrally on the string above the end of my bed. During the night I watched this picture of orange pansies slowly crawl snail-like along the string, first to the left, then to the right, as if trying to escape. The most surreal moment was on the previous morning. My hair was standing on end, my face swollen like a melon, drains attached to my neck, a fat breathing tube down my throat, a feeding tube in my nose. A doctor I had never seen before came across. He leaned over my bed, smiled, and said very distinctly: 'Good morning, Madam.' For one moment I panicked: had I had the wrong operation? I made a sort of approximate male noise and he got the message. Reminded of George IV's exclamation when told that Napoleon was dead: 'Is she, by God!' Tempted to use *Call Me Madam* as the title for this book.

Phlegm isn't an issue you want to dwell on, but after several days on your back, and profoundly weak, it becomes a major problem. Left temporarily deaf, my breath, especially at night, sounds to me like thunder, and I feel that the rattling in my lungs with every exhaled breath must be shaking the walls and keeping others awake. In the night, fearful of not being able to breathe, I wake in panic, thinking I am drowning. I have an oxygen mask, but it's one-size-for-all and a bad fit.

The surgeons visit twice a day and seem happy. They use a Doppler machine, the size and shape of a Walkman, to test if the 'flap' (the newly modelled jaw) has taken. It's placed in my open mouth, and moved slowly across the new flap, and we all listen intently. If there is a soft surging sound, then the blood is beginning to flow. What is now dead white will, hopefully, over the months, take on the pink of mouth-flesh, though it will remain swollen for a long while. Only when it has finally settled shall I be fitted with new teeth.

On the fourth day, in the evening, I'm moved out of Intensive Care to the less traumatic environment of a ward. But I've contracted an MRSA infection in the neck wound, so am shuttled into a small side room, plus loo. Today the hospital has been upped by the Government from two stars to three; Southampton reduced from two stars to one. So glad I chose Salisbury for all sorts of reasons. Don't feel like any visitors. Not allowed out of bed yet ...

27th July

... until this morning. Very wobbly, but move to chair for a couple of hours. Full team of surgeons/doctors visit. They are so impressive and very encouraging. Can't read anything yet, nor watch television. Listen to music.

28th July

The most wretched night so far. The hallucinations seem to get worse. I'm fed with a thick milky fluid, wired up to a feeder. Up many times in the night: each occasion involves buzzing for the night sister, getting unhooked and switching off the machine, being helped to the loo, being helped back again, being re-attached, with much sorting out and sticking on of various wires. In between come the waking hallucinations: walls covered with fine manuscript writing, written on the slant, which I can't quite read without glasses; the ceiling slowly descending towards me, walls flapping, corners full of ants, spiders and the occasional green mouse; the sound of people talking about me but just out of earshot. Hyperventilating, the heart racing. At 2 a.m. begin to think I'm going mad. Sit up and for three hours try to be rational: hold a wooden cross in my hands and repeat my mantras and Psalm 139. Nothing works. Feel, for the first time, a real sense of desolation. Only in the morning do I understand that this is the effect of the morphine. But by then I have persuaded myself that I've been taking part in a film, that I've had enough, and certainly don't want this feeding tube up my nose. So I pull it out with immense satisfaction, though rather surprised by its length ...

29th July

... and at 7.30 a.m. I telephone A. to say I've done so, and please may I come home? Doctors not best pleased. Dr M. and I very slowly insert new feeding-tube.

Long wait for X-ray to discover if it's made its way into the lungs (bad) or stomach (good). Luckily we've got it right. Sit out of bed for a few hours: still totally weak. Surreal night:

the sister is surprised to come in for change of feed at 2 a.m. to find me immovable, my pyjamas removed and tied in knots, the wires from my feeder imprisoning me. During the day my face begins to change shape: great jowls appear, a hard, ridged, pendulous neck, a lump of a chin. Dr M. a bit concerned at late-evening visit: 'If it's any worse at your midnight and 2 a.m. feeds we may have to take you back to theatre and do some draining.' Returns with doctor in operating gear. Prefers to wait until morning. Dream that it's been proved by an American court that I've been palmed off with someone else's face, and that by the morning I shall find mine restored just as it was. Deeply disappointed to discover on waking that this is a lie. But face no worse.

30th July

A. visits daily at 11, 2.30 and 7.30. She walks Camas by the Avon each morning at 6.45, which proves therapeutic: still summer mornings, a faint mist on the deserted river, occasional glimpses of the kingfisher. This p.m. she wheels me outside and I try a few halting, exhausting steps. Face still grossly swollen: shouldn't like to meet in the dark the creature I see in the mirror. Being fed on liquid through tubes and isolated, so that even the usual hospital round of meals and the variety of comings and goings on the ward aren't there to break the routine. Attention fairly spasmodic: a few nurses become immediate favourites. Strange how you know at once who is a natural and has the touch. Feeling of desperate activity on the ward today (Sunday): 16 people await operations, mostly damaged limbs. Some have waited two days. My feeding machine packs up during the night: bleeps loudly each time I doze off. Endless succession of nurses try their hand at mending it. Fail.

31st July

Young, attractive woman doctor comes at 7.15. Would I like a shower? Yes: it's aggressively hot. Wait two hours: no blood pressure or temperature taken, feeding machine still defunct. Ward still spinning, by the sound of it. Get up shakily and attempt shower. A mistake: I nearly faint and just make it back to bed. New feeding dispenser arrives at 12.30. A. was told yesterday that for every minute of anaesthetic, it takes you a day to get over it. Reckon I had at least fifteen hours, which suggests some three years ... which *must* be wrong! Apparently most insurance firms won't pay up if you have an accident driving within a year of a major op. Sounds more likely.

Pointlessly, they bring me a daily menu. Not too tempted by today's alternative to the endless drip of the intravenous sticky fluid: puréed corned beef hash. A bit feverish tonight. Feel low: such a long haul ahead. Time ceases to mean much. 'About four days ago ...' I begin, and am corrected, 'No, that was yesterday.' Listen to Tallis's *Spem in Alium* (Winchester Cathedral Choir).

Complications. Start passing blood just before A. leaves. Suspected bladder infection. Dr M. comes and prescribes immediate antibiotic. None of this type in ward and pharmacy closed. Into my deep midnight sleep my favourite night sister comes like a conspirator, shakes me awake, and says triumphantly that she has found some in another patient's locker: grinds it up and feeds it intravenously. Wake hourly. Assessed in morning as merely a post-catheter problem, but antibiotics, once started, must continue to the bitter end.

1st August

Various doctors come. Lab. reports on lymph glands not yet received. Some of clips removed from around neck wound: sore and unpleasant. How quickly the outside world fades, each detail here carrying its own comforting or challenging overtones, the ward never still, day or night. Meanwhile the world continues unawares: suffering, wrote Auden, takes place 'while someone else is eating or opening a window or just walking dully along ...'[8] Woken from a snooze for immediate transfer into main ward. Wheeled in bed, my

72

alter ego (the feeder) trailing behind, into the mixed ward. Five minutes later a slightly ruffled nurse swabs me for MRSA, then I'm smartly whipped back to my small room. It was a mistake: I'm still infectious. A ten-minute diversion in a non-eventful day. I.D. comes and explains that I picked up an MRSA infection in Intensive Care, but they failed to swab me again. Suspect hospital is pretty jumpy on this issue, and not communicating as well as in other areas.

Patientline, personal TV, radio and mobile by each bed, looks good but is untrustworthy. 'What do you want to know about radio?' it asks. I press an innocuous-looking button: 'The page you have asked for is unobtainable' it tells me, 'as it contains language which some may find offensive.'

2nd August
Restless night. Fall into deep sleep at 7 a.m. to be woken 30 minutes later by two doctors and Bishop P., just off to the States. Not at my best. Followed by two unknown doctors, curious to inspect new mouth. Must endure them trying the Doppler machine to listen to the blood pulsing in the 'flap', though it's increasingly tender. More blood tests. Pain-killers and antibiotics injected into the tube taped across forehead. Somewhere, on some remote computer, all this is being co-ordinated.

Colin Semper writes to ask if the prayer of friends and loved ones has helped/is helping? Immediate response: in the run-up to the operation and since, 'Yes, hugely and comfortingly, in the sense of feeling valued and affirmed.' 'By love enfolded' has to be translated into the reality of each community, each individual. 'There is nothing that makes us love a man so much as praying for him,' wrote William Law. Only in people can the compassionate love of God be incarnated and expressed. For most of the time I'm too weak to pray for myself and am utterly dependent on others, whether for bed-baths or for consciously holding me in God's presence, and asking that this cancer may be used creatively. Must tease this out further. I brought in

Celebrating Common Prayer (the Franciscan version of the Offices used daily for morning prayer in the cathedral), but haven't the energy to use it yet.

I.D. comes again. Explains that the very long anaesthetic badly affected the liver enzymes, but the blood is normalising. Glad something is. A. brings in a mass of cards and letters. Wheels me outside for some fresh air: the far fields a welcome sight as they catch the light of a thin sun. Can't settle for long at anything: a chapter of a novel, a Louis Armstrong/Ella Fitzgerald tape, a little writing. Listening to the audiotape of Jill Balcon reading Claire Tomalin's *Samuel Pepys*. Tonight at 9, nurse P. has just unplugged my feeding tube to insert medication before hurrying away at sound of shouting. For next hour all nurses coping with emergency, but (unplugged) my feeder continues its relentless course of expelling sticky liquid, and P. returns to find me awash in it. Cleaned up, and rewarded by being allowed to pass the night unplugged from the feeder.

3rd August

Overhear nurse temporarily on loan from a long-term medical (as opposed to surgical) ward: 'It's a relief to get away from all that endless crying.' Much of it, I guess, the emotional pain when faced with long-term or terminal illness, with which hospices cope so much better than hospitals. Visit from cancer care team: they seem happy. Listen to Fats Waller. In p.m. wheeled by non-communicative student to Oral Clinic, where L. removes rest of stubborn neck staples. I.D. present but a bit spaced out and anxious – not about me, but about a house purchase – and receives call telling him he has 15 minutes to complete the deal. Very weary on return to bed. Watch the Gielgud/Jeremy Irons scene from *Brideshead Revisited*. A. tells me those amazing swifts have gone. Birds which can roost on the wing, some have been shown to live as long as 20 years, flying 500 miles a day, amounting in their lifetime (unless slaughtered over Italy or Spain) to as much as 3.8 million miles. In his poem

'Haymaking', Edward Thomas says they look 'as if the bow had blown off with the arrow'.

4th August

Still on feeder, but allowed lumpy porridge for breakfast. A sort of milestone in this narrowed world of hospital. Write brief cards to the three religious communities that are supporting me: West Malling, Tymawr and Burford. Forced to drink three litres of water a day and keep a written account. Revolting puréed cauliflower for lunch. Supper not much better: potato soup, roast chicken, chocolate mousse: all reduced to a thin gruel. Lovely flowers arrive from Patricia Routledge: a bouquet from Hyacinth Bucket (a.k.a. Bouquet). So drugged at night now that I'm unaware of nurses coming in small hours to 'flush out' feeding tube.

5th August

I.D. comes early: swabs reveal that MRSA still active, though wounds seem to be healing. But it means yet another antibiotic. ('We don't often give that for MRSA,' says a puzzled nurse later, unhelpfully.) I.D. wants me to stay in over the weekend while they monitor food and drink. A. has learned how to text. Received one from Sarah, on holiday in Eastern Europe, enthusing about glories of Budapest. Sent one back: 'Dad now on puréed food.' Such are our changed priorities. Visited by R., the one-to-one nurse who (I'm told) looked after me so impressively early on in Intensive Care: 'I wanted to meet you properly, because even though you couldn't speak you still tried to thank me each time I did anything nasty to you.' They forget my supper. Finally rustle up a packet of powdered tomato soup. Everything tastes the same: medicinal and sweet and strangely *pink*. Long for the sharp tastes again.

I.D. comes. All biopsy results have come back. Flesh surrounding the tumour is now clear, as are the glands and almost all lymph nodes. However, the cancer has begun to spread to those on the left-hand side beneath the ear and, if left, will slowly creep down as if descending a ladder. This will mean six weeks of radiotherapy in Southampton. We both instinctively knew it. A. looks so weary tonight. Believe one night-nurse thinks me fussy. Rather fierce and unsmiling for the past couple of nights. Tonight see large creature on door: is it real or have the hallucinations returned? Ask her. She picks up a book and slams it dead. Pats me on the leg as she leaves. Minor breakthrough.

6th August

Have asked for medication nightly at 8.30 so that I can get to sleep. Can't buck the system. It continues to come some time after 10 when I've just fallen asleep. Breakfast arrives in ward at 8.15: get mine (three fruit juices and a yoghurt) at 9.20. Doctor assures me new swab taken last week: know it wasn't and prove to be right. Getting more critical: sign of longing for home. Listen to Pepys for an hour first thing each day. Says that he 'admired his doctors as much for their conversation as their skills'. Feel the same about I.D. who today removes feeding tube and promises home on Monday. Reading outstanding novel: Sue Gee's *The Mysteries of Glass*. Slow, perceptive, wonderful descriptions of natural world. Saturday *Guardian* good as ever, but heavy fare for hospital.

What must I explore further when I'm home? How far the enduring melody of my faith, the sense of being held by God at the deepest level of my being, has made a difference. Yeats wrote in a different context of how 'things fall apart; the centre cannot hold'. Need to discover if and how the centre holds when your life temporarily falls apart, and what that centre may be. Was it possible to find some sane central core during the worst of the delusions? What, if anything, have I learned about myself and the community of prayer and what now *really* matters in my life? I'm still not thinking very clearly. A. says that during the days and nights when I was deluded it was quite frightening and gave her just a small insight into the pain of one whose partner has developed Alzheimer's. The person you know so intimately is no longer there.

When I read the night office, Compline, in the light of the madness of last week, the words, 'From evil dreams defend our eyes,/ From nightly fears and fantasies' take on a new significance.

The most inspired touch has come from Christina Shewell in Bristol: a couple of postcards each day containing between one and five brightly coloured words, the cards arriving in a random but still logical order for me to make up into a sentence. By now I have put them in my chosen order:

> I AM/ BELOVED ON THE EARTH/ HOLDING ON IN THERE/ BUT/ I CAN SEE/ LIGHT IN THE DARK/ THERE WILL BE/ HEALING/ THAT PERFECT CUP OF TEA/ SOMETIMES LIKE MOVING THROUGH TREACLE/ BUT ALSO/ WONDER NONETHELESS/ LEARNING TO DANCE AGAIN/ GLORY BE/ PRAYER FLAG IN THE WIND/ STILL SMALL VOICE/ EVER-LASTING ARMS/ A JOY FOR EVER.

Many have come as open postcards straight to the ward, and (through my ever-open door) I've enjoyed the bewildered expression on the face of the ward clerk each morning as she reads a single, seemingly meaningless phrase. Regarded me in a very strange way when I tried to explain.

7th August
So, fingers crossed, I'll be home tomorrow. There have been gains and losses: *came in with* malignant tumour in centre of lower jaw which would certainly have spread and proved to be the end of me; *go out with* newly constructed bottom jaw, pillow of flesh from thigh under tongue, all but two end teeth gone, very swollen and numb face, protruding lower lip, scar from ear to ear and MRSA still active in wound, long scar on thigh, bruised and tender chest, numb and tender left ear and shoulder, signs of cancer spreading from one lymph node. Could be much worse. I also have a new

admiration for the sheer professionalism of the cancer care team and the skill and care I've received. And, given a few more months, the hope of many more years of a life which will almost certainly be changed, but will once again be rich and fulfilling.

My Communion brought by a woman somewhat flustered by being forced to wear a plastic apron and rubber gloves before approaching me. A new experience, apparently, for us both. Watch thrilling last two hours of second Test Match: amazing last wicket stand. We win by two runs. Saddened by sudden death of Robin Cook. Thought him prickly and awkward when he was on a CND panel I chaired at Cambridge, but his recent stand on matters of principle has been important to our political life; there are few such healthily disruptive politicians left. I.D. comes. Diana is visiting and asks him to explain exactly what he's done to me. He takes 15 minutes to draw and describe it: D. greatly impressed. Mark and Joanie come down from London, *en route* for Brittany in the morning.

8th August

Long to be home in own bed and have a bath again. It's been a bumpy ride: much of it anticipated, some (fortunately) not. Warned once again that I may feel 'mini-bereavement' when the snug womb of hospital is no longer there and may become irritable and/or depressed. R.D., the plastic surgeon whose voice thankfully prevailed at the operation in opting for a graft from my leg rather than my wrist, comes to say goodbye. Apart from the hiccough of two returns to theatre, says I've done exceptionally well. Final X-ray of mouth at 11, then four-hour wait for pharmacists' pills and gallons of pink Fortifresh, a farewell to the nurses, and home. Beautiful day: trees and garden flowers extra-brilliant after 15 days of muted interiors. Immediately fall asleep.

9th August

Very feeble. Shave tentatively where I can. Neck ridged like a potato field. Read through 300-plus cards and letters. Flowers from Salisbury Playhouse (where I'm chaplain): they've been so thoughtful throughout. Still very sore in unexpected places, and tonight spectacular bruising is emerging in shades of yellow and purple. Many parts numb: in others, when touched, a sense of pins and needles and what nurse L. calls 'spiders crawling over your skin'. It's going to be a long haul; but I'm alive!

10th August

Further card from C.: 'EVEN AN OCCASIONAL SPARKLE'. Wake often in night, heart racing. With A.'s help, manage first tentative bath, and wash hospital away. She sensibly rations me to writing one card, and making one phone call a day. Voice sounds as if mouth full of stones. Doctors have warned repeatedly what a very slow process recovery will be. Must anticipate the continuing weakness and discomfort and learn (as with M.E.) to live one day at a time, and be 'glad in it', grateful for small kindnesses, the garden with its changing light, colours, birds; and the daily gift of life.

Reflecting on God (2)

This is the real test: that of patience, humour, trust and hope. They can only flourish in a climate of acceptance, a recognition of the value to be found in the willingness to wait, wholly dependent on the matching willingness of those who love you to serve you in Blake's 'minute particulars' of love. God *is* in the cancer and its treatment, not plainly but in subtle, hidden, interpersonal ways, and much effortless, book-learned 'God-language' that trips so easily off the tongue may mask or distort this fundamental truth. The truth that the grace of God may be scented, and must be sought for, in human words and actions, daily incarnated in the actions of those made in his likeness. That could be to diminish and domesticate God, but not if you hold it in tandem with the knowledge that ours is a God who must constantly be sought for and waited upon – R. S. Thomas's experience of the Presence who seems to have departed from the space just as you enter it, the elusive Other. God perceived as what my lifelong friend Hugh Dickinson calls

> a sort of residual movement in the air ... Perhaps it is like homeopathy, God diluted to barely molecular essences but able nevertheless to affect us imperceptibly by becoming incorporated into us. I'm sure there is a humanity in God long before the appearance of *homo sapiens* – anything even faintly hominoid is *capax Dei* (has a capacity for God) to some degree. Us he can inhabit fully, and in so doing endures and groans and travails as part of the deal; including our despair. But something gets born in the darkness I know, something of which I become aware only much later, when to my own surprise I find I am changed. Sheer gift, unplanned, unexpected, undeserved. I suppose that's what they mean by grace?[9]

In the same letter, he writes of an

> awareness of the Divine in us ... an intense engagement with the Divine Love somewhere at the root of our being ... If that is so of our aware moments I suppose it must be so of our blind and dark times – perhaps more so. I can't pretend I actually feel it; but sometimes after the groaning is over I have been aware that there has been a dark glory around.

A 'dark glory'. Michael Ramsey, who was always strong on 'glory', would have admired the phrase.

No, I can't pretend that I actually feel it either, so what do I say to Colin when he writes, 'What I shall want to know in the fulness of time is: Did you feel *held* – or is it something people say?' (As in Sr Pia's letter to me: 'May God enfold you in his love – and may you know it.') Yes, I felt held, right up to the morning of the operation, enfolded in love; but in the dark days that followed I felt nothing at times but the darkness (as Jesus – though I draw back from making the analogy – felt the darkness of desolation in the Garden of

Gethsemane and, for a while, on the Cross). That is part of the human experience. But what I *felt* is hardly relevant, for the 'feelings' were caused by the poison in my veins. The reality is that I was not losing my reason; that I was vigorously upheld in God's presence; and in retrospect I find that not only the truth but the greatest comfort.

These are matters which loom large when you are at the margins, mysteries to which there are no slick answers. So when C. asks: 'Was God absent?' the answer is both 'yes' (absent to me, for I couldn't sense him), and 'no' (for others were affirming my value in his sight and acting as channels for his love). And both are true. After all, it's the poetry, not the bare bones, of the divine story that offers the necessary home to ambiguity. The ambiguity of the divine absence, the *via negativa*, the mystic's 'deep but dazzling darkness', and the reality of the indwelling Spirit.

Greatly enjoying Julian Barnes' *Arthur and George*. Watch Chaplin's *A Dog's Life* before early bed.

11th August
Take painkillers only at night now. Feel totally gummed-up. A. is producing thoughtful puréed food: apparently same helpings as hers but reduced to half the size. Three final cards from Christina: 'A THING OF BEAUTY' and 'QUIET WRITING'; and to sign off, 'LOVE'. She and Mark come to lunch. Knowing my passion for the sea, C. brings large bottle of sea-water from Ringstead Bay. Pour it into washing-up bowl and I sit in the sun and paddle. House stuffed with gifts of flowers: white and purple orchids, red and yellow roses, white hydrangea, sunflowers and larkspur, pinks and freesias, agapanthus and chrysanthemums. Prayer life still a bit hit-and-miss. Lack of any energy affects that too. Shall associate past three weeks with the scent of sweet-peas, a small vase of them constantly beside my bed. Best to be ill in the summer.

12th August

To hospital at 9.30. Pleased with progress. But no MRSA results. They finally believe me that I've not been swabbed again, even though L., the clinic sister, took the kit to the ward ten days ago. Overlooked. Ask (as joke) if the flesh from the thigh now in my mouth will continue to grow hairs? 'Oh, yes.' Help! Daily lunch diet: home-made soup, half a mashed avocado with *creme fraiche*, a mashed banana. Best tastes yet. Diana comes with wild marjoram from Martin Down, Pam Waller with raspberries. A. was saying to them both how strongly she felt supported by the raft of prayer in recent weeks; of how words can't explain it. It is (in George Herbert's words) 'something understood': i.e. experienced instinctively, not capable of any logical reasoning in imprecise and stumbling words, but – like love, like grace – *given* and accepted without question.

Understand a bit better the way doctors must handle the predictability/unpredictability factor in a major operation or illness. I knew exactly what the surgeons expected to do (though in the event they changed it) and what they predicted it would be like afterwards. But the *unpredictable* factor is the unique self who is the patient, with our differing reactions to this massive invasion of the self's territory, our own history, emotions, pain toleration, dream pattern, hopes and fears. These will not only affect the rate of recovery, but the inner experience of the sickness. It is my operation and my cancer: *like* that of others but just that crucial bit *unlike* too. All very obvious, and a good surgeon will no doubt assess the patient as to how anxious they are and how much should be revealed. (I remember one of the Southampton doctors telling me to look him in the eye, and silently hold his gaze.)

Watch the Third Test: becoming hooked on cricket in my old age. Some liquidised pork for supper, followed by some crushed Rennies. Up every couple of hours in night. Dream of Great Aunt Maggie, dead these 60 years, and never consciously thought of since. Extraordinary the people who take up residence in your head.

13th August

Feel able at last to say short morning office. The Psalms are extraordinary, always appropriate whatever your state, as apt for your wedding day as your funeral. Set Psalm today is 31:7–end:

> I will rejoice and be glad because of your mercy,
> for you have seen my affliction; you know my distress ...
> You have set my feet in an open place.
> Blessed is the Lord!
> for he has shown me the wonders of his love ...

Lesson not so helpful: the imminent second coming of the Son of Man; one of the issues on which Jesus, man of his time, went with the popular view and got it wrong. Early each morning flocks of finches, tits and sparrows sweep through the garden, briefly de-bugging the apple tree. Throat wound has swollen more and is uncomfortable, leaving me anxious that the MRSA is increasingly infecting the wound. A wet, difficult evening, helped by phone calls from the family in Prague.

14th August

Up hourly till 4, then dream I'm serving delicious puréed meals in very upper-class Women's Institute. Forced by female version of Gordon Ramsay to paint all the plates first, which is annoyingly time-consuming, and find his/her swearing tiresome. Shaving – getting dressed – exhausting. Morning Psalm 90:

> The span of our life is seventy years,
> perhaps in strength even eighty;
> yet the sum of them is but labour and sorrow,
> for they pass away quickly and we are gone ...
> So teach us to number our days
> that we may apply our hearts to wisdom.

Listen to Radio 4 Sunday morning service: my old BBC friend Ian Mackenzie from Edinburgh. Wise, imaginative, enviably good. A reflection on the arts and spirituality based on his life-changing experience, aged 17, at the first Edinburgh Festival in 1947, held in the wake of the Holocaust and of a war ended by the horror of Hiroshima and Nagasaki. 'The human spirit had faced, but not resolved, the enigmas of beauty versus obscenity, truth versus distortion.'[10] Speaks of a performance of Bach's *B Minor Mass* 'as Malcolm Sargent whipped the Huddersfield Choir up that mountain of hope and over the summit'; of a concert given by Bruno Walter conducting his beloved Vienna Philharmonic, three years after Hitler had cut a great swathe through the Jews in the orchestra; of how they played the waltzes of Strauss, many of the musicians swaying to the rhythm but some with tears pouring down their faces. 'Tread softly, for you tread on my nightmares. I had a fleeting vision of a God who has entrusted to the human race the fathomless mysteries of free will,' and of 'a middle Eastern carpenter who has decided to dance for the human race into the dark'. Describes a mind-blowing concert in the Usher Hall: Verdi's *Requiem*, orchestra and chorus of La Scala, Milan conducted by Victor de Sabata. The sheer overwhelming power of the *Dies Irae*, the Day of Wrath, the Judgement. The Festival was devised to be a celebration of the human spirit, including the dark side of humanity. Here were experiences of darkness and redemption. Reeling out of the Hall, Ian climbed Blackford Hill and walked for hours, the lights of Edinburgh far below. Suddenly he felt a sense of

God silently embracing the world, and myself as one small but living part of it ... God embracing everything, transcending our carefully wired-up categories. He affirmed who and what we are and what we are doing here. Not since that night have I found a wider truth, a deeper magic, a firmer presence. And art brought it home to me, or me to it ... I'd begun learning to open myself up to other dimensions. All part of a rhythm born in the stars. A rhythm of love.

Judy Rees comes for tea with Vikram Seth. He sent me a card in hospital with a green leaf curled inside it. Tell him it reminded me of Chesterton's words: 'There is but one sin, to call the green leaf grey,' and of my hallucinatory green mice. He brings us the first copy of his soon-to-be-published new book, *Two Lives*, and inscribes it: 'To M. and A. May your green leaves never appear grey, only your grey mice green.' Perplexing for any who may come across it in years to come. He is remarkable, both as a writer and as a human being: witty, acutely observant, generous, with a passion for the poetry of George Herbert, in whose house he is now living. Describes himself as 'a quasi-agnostic Hindu', but the carpenter of Nazareth would have warmed to him.

Third Test exciting. But the days are long, and I feel stuck. Afternoons are worst. They warned me that it would now all slow down. But I'm here, surrounded by books and care. Must dig deep for patience. Watch the Prom: Mozart and Mahler's First, played by a remarkable orchestra, the West-Eastern Divan Orchestra, founded by Daniel Barenboim, a Jew, and the late Edward Said, a Palestinian, and made up of young Jews and Arabs to prove that music, with a power far beyond that of language, has the power to heal and reconcile and speak across all the barriers of prejudice and frozen history. As Barenboim reiterated tonight, it is the ability to compose, perform, and listen to music that makes us most human. Next week they play in Ramallah on the West Bank; and tomorrow the Israelis are starting to pull out of the Gaza Strip. In their important book of conversations, *Parallels and Paradoxes*,[11] Barenboim tells of a Syrian boy who had never met an Israeli, and was brought up to fear and hate them – until he found himself sharing a music-stand with an Israeli cellist. He argues that music, together with theatre and opera, over and above providing comfort and entertainment, has a social purpose. It may ask disturbing questions of both performer and listener. In totalitarian societies it was the only place where political ideas could be criticised.

A performance of Beethoven, under the Nazis or under any kind of totalitarian regime, whether left or right, suddenly assumes the call for freedom, even becomes a direct criticism of the policies of the regime and therefore, is actually a much more disturbing and ... uplifting thing.[12]

Said agrees:

Beethoven's music, and particularly the fantastic Choral Symphony, is all about a certain kind of affirmation (and connects) to the affirmation of the human being in society, with promises of fulfilment, of liberation, and brotherhood ... All the positive things we want to say about human existence are (contained) explicitly ... in the last movement, but implicitly in this fantastic stream of pulsating, organically connected music, which seems to say, 'The human adventure is worth it in some way' ... You have a sense that Beethoven is sustained by an abiding, rational faith ... in humanity.[13]

15th August

Often dream of the theatre. Tonight I'm cast as Romeo in a production in a London comprehensive school. My Juliet is a rather dumpy 14-year-old. Realise I could be her great-grandfather, but this doesn't seem to have occurred to them, so don't point it out. Morning Psalm 130: 'I wait for the Lord; my soul waits for him; in his word is my hope.'

Good letter from Stuart, Prior of Burford: 'I have never known the community so united in its prayerful concern as it was on the day of your operation.' Which moves me to tears. Dear God, I feel weak! Parts of me – face, jaw, neck – are still numb; parts – chest, shoulder, 12-inch wound on thigh – would be less tender if they were as numb as the former. Nick and Elizabeth Tyndall call in *en route* for Dorset. N. asks me:

'How are you?'
'I could be worse.'
'How?'

'I could be dead.'

'That might be rather better.'

Can't decide if they mean it. (*Later:* Nick knew then, as I didn't, that he had cancer. Two months later he learnt that it was terminal. He died with great courage on Easter Monday, having said a grateful and gracious farewell to all the members of his family.)

I've never been wholly persuaded by Paul's vacillating (in his letter to the Philippians) about whether it were better to go on living, for there is more work to do, or to depart and be 'with Christ'. He says that though we carry death with us in our bodies we never cease to be confident:

> For to me life is Christ, and death gain ... Which then shall I choose? I cannot tell. I am torn two ways: what I should like is to depart and be with Christ, that is better by far; but for your sake there is greater need for me to stay on in the body.[14]

To want to hold onto this God-given life for as long as we can is a deeply human instinct, and does nothing to lessen the truth that in death as in life we are in a relationship with our Christlike Creator that transcends this material body. The first we experience daily: the other we cannot imagine. John Robinson ended his final sermon with these words:

> According to my chronology (Paul) lived nearly ten years after writing those words: others would say it was shorter. But how little does it matter. He had passed beyond time and its calculations. He had risen with Christ.[15]

From bed watch the low half-moon, gradually turning orange as it sinks to the horizon behind the thin, illuminated spire of the distant cathedral.

16th August

Wake in panic at 12.30, lungs blocked, finding it hard to breathe. Coughing simply aggravates the swollen throat.

Interesting how an excess of mucus membrane becomes the source of one of the Elizabethan 'humours', identifying you as 'phlegmatic': i.e. 'cool, calm, sluggish, apathetic'. Don't recognise much of a match there. The Elizabethans were simply following the teaching of Galen, born in the second century AD. His belief was that the patient was suffering from an imbalance of the four elements of earth, air, fire and water with the four cardinal humours of the body (blood, phlegm, bile and black bile). This was to be a view of disease that dominated medicine until the start of the nineteenth century. We still speak of rheumatism (too much water), pyrexia or fever (too much fire), pneumonia (not enough air), cholera (too much bile), and melancholia (too much black bile). The Chinese have had for close on 2000 years a similar scheme based on the imbalance of *yin* and *yang*, in the force known as *chi*. For them and their doctors, the body is a series of energy conduits. *Chi*, the name of this energy, flows along systematic meridians. They don't coincide with any known physiological structures as in Western medicine – physical or chemical abnormalities – but rather with hidden forces which are out of balance. They describe their task as 'restoring secret harmonies'. They see acupuncture as intervening in an energy system. The same is true of their use of herbs. Also, massaging the body's pressure points (as in reflexology) helps to get the energy flowing again. Incidentally, Chinese physicians only received a fee if their patients remained in good health. Their task was to 'stay healthy by living correctly; temperament, diet, thoughts, emotions, and exercise were all important in a system in which the patient took primary responsibility for sickness or health'.[16]

For the Elizabethans (see Shakespeare *passim*), our make-up is not only influenced by the stars (the popularity of astrology shows that many still think so), but by the four humours or elements which corresponded to what, in the days before the discovery of the Periodic Table, they thought of as the four natural elements: *earth* – cold and dry =

melancholy; *water* – cold and moist = phlegm; *air* – hot and moist = blood; *fire* – hot and dry = choler. They believed that food is made of these four elements, that it passes through the stomach to the liver, which converts it into four liquid substances, the humours. In using the words 'temperament' or 'complexion' they meant the tempering of one humour by another, or the intertwining of the humours to create character. The noblest people, and therefore the most healthy, had the four humours in a fine balance. Cleopatra claims she is 'all air and fire'. Certainly she's a 'hot property', but unbalanced. In Brutus, claimed Mark Antony, the humours were mixed just right:

> This was the noblest Roman of them all ...
> His life was gentle, and the elements
> So mix'd in him that nature could stand up
> And say to all the world, 'This was a man!'

So much for phlegm in the night.

In the morning Jeremy Davies comes from the cathedral and celebrates Communion: all the priests here, thank God, are first and foremost gifted pastors. We are spoiled for choice. An hour later L. phones from the Oral Clinic to say that it's 'not good news'; the swab shows MRSA still active in the neck. We're confused. I.D. said that if the infection really took hold it could be a serious setback. He is on holiday and another consultant says 'do nothing' until my visit at end of week. On an impulse, A. drives to the busy Clinic, waits 10 minutes and is then seen for 45 minutes by L., cancer care team sister. She says:

(i) The infection may last some time, but the wound is not open and they hope the body's immune system will deal with it. But I may carry it for the rest of my life.

(ii) Between four and eight weeks is a most difficult time, a new stage, when all the body's natural healing channels begin slowly to assert themselves after the massive assault of the operation. The two saliva glands under the tongue having been removed, the other glands are working overtime to restore normality. 'If he had seen what had been done to him in the operating theatre, he'd understand a bit more how he was feeling.'

(iii) She spelled out the different levels of anxiety (conscious and unconscious) which have built up, from the first suggestion of something seriously wrong, through the biopsy, the weeks of waiting, the immediate pre-operation days, the days following. You lurch from one thing to the next, never really having the time or energy to deal with any of them, and have to come to terms with the significance of an altered life as the weeks and months go by. From now on, every eruption of the skin, every puzzling lump, will carry the inevitable question: 'cancer?'

(iv) The time has come to stop re-running the operation to everyone who has the patience to listen.

(vi) I should count myself lucky: 25 years ago I would have been left with a large hole in my jaw.

A. comes home reassured. L. is an example of the NHS at its very best.

Watch half of Bogart and Bacall in *The Big Sleep*. Lovely three-quarter moon and calm night.

17th August
Another perfect day. Walking Camas early by the river, A. sees the kingfisher for the third time this week. Boringly predictable day: 7.45 say short morning prayer; 8 breakfast (porridge and yoghurt) in bed; dress slowly. Write a card or two, read the *Independent* and listen to music. Mashed banana at 11. Lunch (soup, puréed avocado, mashed nectarine), then rest and doze until 3.30. Visitor at 4. Yoghurt for tea. Juiced mango at 6. Puréed supper (fish or scrambled egg, veg., ice cream); an hour of TV; gentle bath and bed. Camas a great companion, and thinks my constant presence very thoughtful.

Reflecting on desire

Reading Vikram's *Two Lives*. His Uncle Shanti wrote to him when he was a student: 'I am a great believer that you will get what you want but you must want it and not just wish it.' And V. comments: 'I am still not entirely certain what Uncle meant ... but I often thought about it in the years that followed.' I believe what he meant is what Pia means by her emphasis that in petitionary prayer you must ask yourself one question: 'What do I really *want*?' It's the question I had to learn in my long bout of M.E. 20 years ago. What I finally learned was that I wanted to redeem that experience, to learn from it, to bring good out of it, not as a vague wish but as a deep hunger; and it's the question I was determined should dominate this experience of cancer. It's the distinction between a general, not very well defined wish for healing or happiness or fulfilment, and a deeply focused, engaged and confident *desire and longing* for this one thing, the one thing needful for me to learn at this moment in my life. Having once discovered what I've called the *cantus firmus*, the fixed ground of a lifelong melody which has so far proved enduring, my desire must now be to see how to play new improvisations which are faithful to that melody, one which can embrace the darkness and not find it destructive.

Augustine defined what has struck a chord down the ages as the true and authentic desire of the human heart: that ultimate knowledge of resting in God, for 'Thou hast made us for Thyself and our hearts are restless until they rest in Thee.' The One 'whose promises', in the words of the collect, 'exceed all that we can desire'. I believe that every authentic experience of love and goodness, beauty and truth (hard to define intellectually, but instantly recognisable emotionally) is a reflection of that Divine Ground which beckons to us, even in the dark. 'God in the cancer': God inviting me to grow a little through being at the centre of such dedicated skill and care, kindness and prayer. My deep, instinctive desire is to be free of the cancer, and enjoy to the full the sights and sounds of this extraordinary world for a good

91

many years yet. But that needs to be balanced by an equal desire to simplify my life and find out what matters and what endures when the chips are down.

Certainly I have been forced to face as never before the reality of dying. Not that it is possible to imagine your own death. And maybe, still feeling pretty vulnerable, this is not the moment to go further down that cul-de-sac. For it feels quite scary. If only more people understood that priests are as exposed and human as every other person. As R. S. Thomas writes, to have faith means to live 'somewhere between doubt and certainty'. Christians are in no way protected, and don't have things any easier than non-believers: we're called, rather, to see life against a background of the transcendent sacred – that God-dimension which can't be trapped in words, but in the long history of human experience cannot be denied. Where it is repressed by atheistic regimes it runs on quietly underground. Our human fear of dying doesn't invalidate the Christian belief in resurrection, however unimaginable another form of life may be; but it does make the point that fear of the dark and the unknown are common to us all, and that without such questioning faith, hope and trust would not be as costly or as meaningful as they are. In the light of the Holocaust, the daily violence and scandalous poverty, the death of a loved one, or the secret destructive nature of the cancer cell, hope and trust can be very costly indeed, and cause many to write us off as fools. So be it.

I wrote just now of how experiences of love, goodness, beauty, truth, can't be defined intellectually (to the satisfaction of neurologists, say, or post-modernist literary critics); only experienced emotionally. Why do we dismiss the emotions as of less validity than the intellect? In 1912 D. H. Lawrence was writing:

> My great religion is a belief in the blood, the flesh, as being
> wiser than the intellect. We can go wrong in our minds. But
> what the blood feels, and believes, and says, is always true.

Aldous Huxley, commenting on those words, writes:

> Like Blake, who had prayed to be delivered from 'single vision
> and Newton's sleep': like Keats, who had drunk destruction to
> Newton for having explained the rainbow, Lawrence dis-
> approved of too much knowledge, on the score that it dimin-
> ished men's sense of wonder and blunted their sensitivity to
> the great mystery.[17]

A. takes me on my first drive, up the Woodford valley.
Attempt a 50-yard walk. Flattened by it. Watch the rest of
The Big Sleep. Love the way Bogart, even when kissing Bacall,
keeps his hat on. Listen in bed to late Prom: the music of
Arvo Pärt sung by the superb Estonian Philharmonic
Chamber Choir, who sang here in June at the Festival.

18th August

Scanning through the paper, I read of the murder of Brother
Roger of Taizé. Suddenly find myself weeping. Aged 90,
Roger has been knifed in the throat while in the Church of
Reconciliation, sitting (as I have seen him many times)
surrounded by children. Can't bear to think of the trauma
for those children. Tens of thousands of people will be
mourning worldwide one of the great figures of our time.
I've been lucky enough to spend time with a number of
renowned people. Five stand out from the rest for their
powerful, charismatic presence: Nelson Mandela, Mother
Teresa, the Dalai Lama, Desmond Tutu, and – by no means
least – Brother Roger. Like all of us Roger had his weaknesses,
but they faded in the light of his manifest goodness. He had
the most amazing eyes. His face radiated what I could only
call 'Christlikeness', and his luminous smile conveyed a
simplicity and a transparency that to me was akin to what
people mean when they say of Iona that it's a place where
the veil between heaven and earth is a little thinner. In 1974
two of us went to Taizé for a week to make a programme for
BBC Radio 4. Two meetings with Brother Roger were
unforgettable, the first of them in his modest bed-sitting-

room. He wore, as always, his white habit. On three sides were great windows overlooking the Burgundian country-side, their shutters flung wide and the April sun streaming in. The furniture was simply crafted white wood. The room shone. His face lit up when he spoke of those things that lay at his heart: the grace of sharing, of reconciliation and for-giveness, of joy, of the importance of listening to others and the power of music and silence; of the need to live in the present moment and of experiences of resurrection. That night he invited us to join a dozen of the brothers in a small refectory for a simple supper. We sat at one side of a long table, ate without speaking, and listened to the music of Bach. It was one of the best, most meaningful meals of my life. Unforgettable. A kind of Eucharist.

No doubt my tears this morning were not just for Roger and the terrible irony of a violent death in the place of reconciliation, or for the terrible sickness of mind that causes such irrational cries for help. No doubt they were also for A. and me, a necessary part of coming to terms with these past weeks, triggered by real grief at the death of this good and holy man. It says he took a few minutes to die, and that he signalled to the nearest brother that the music and the act of worship should continue. And in his last moments of consciousness I am sure he would have forgiven his attacker. At his funeral requiem his chosen successor as prior, Brother Alois, used this prayer:

> God of greatness, we entrust to your forgiveness Luminata Solcan who, in a moment of sickness, put an end to the life of Brother Roger. With Christ on the cross we say to you: Father, forgive her, for she does not know what she did.

There's an Indian proverb: 'Religion, Patience, Friend and Wife are to be tested at the time of adversity.' For me (so far) the latter two have come through with flying colours; the first two still to be fully tested. Sit in the garden watching the bees bother the lavender and reading V.'s fine book, a loving tribute to his one-armed dentist uncle and his

German Jewish aunt, her mother and sister victims of the Holocaust. A. has driven to Herefordshire for the burial of her mother's ashes. In the evening watch Rogers and Astaire in *Top Hat*, beautifully nostalgic and undemanding.

19th August
Clinic at 9. Pleased with progress, especially with the mouth 'flap' (the new transplant of part of the lower jaw), now fully sealed. Swabbed again for MRSA.

Reflecting on wonder (1)
During the morning a handsome black, white and scarlet Great Spotted woodpecker spends ten minutes de-bugging the dead apple tree. Only second time we have seen one in nine years, his visits almost as rare as those small moments of epiphany when 'God comes, as I had always known/ he would come, unannounced/ remarkable merely for the absence of clamour'.[18] He's very beautiful, with his black head and coral-coloured nape, and makes my day. Chaucer calls him 'woodwale', surviving in some parts still as 'woodwall'. For Andrew Marvell he was 'the hewel' and he writes of how he walks upright on the tree:

> Measuring the Timber with his Foot,
> And all the way, to keep it clean,
> He with his beak, examines well
> Which fit to stand and which to fell.
>
> The good he numbers up, and hacks,
> As if he marked them with the axe.
> But where he, tinkling with his beak,
> Does find the hollow oak to speak,
> That for his building he designs,
> And through the tainted side he mines.
> Who could have thought the tallest oak
> Should fall by such a feeble stroke![19]

What all good scientists share, whether or not they link it to God, is what the poet/astronomer Rebecca Elson (who was to die of cancer at the age of 39) calls in a striking phrase 'a responsibility to awe'. Whichever of Jesus' words and stories may or may not be authentic (as they come to us through the reflections and selection of the Gospel writers and the word-of-mouth tradition circulating among the early Christians), what is beyond dispute is that he had a deep sense of the numinous, a 'responsibilty to awe', a recognition of the Father's life-giving creativity pervading all things. Hugh writes to me of how in all creative art there is 'a radical dependency on a transcendent Other', of how Van Gogh (among many others) saw the natural world as 'seething with divine life'. I've tried to reflect that truth in what I've written elsewhere on the need for a sense of wonder, of the primary human need to give our absorbed attention to whatever (or, more important, whoever) is before us in order to learn to value them. In yesterday's *Guardian* the art critic Tom Lubbock writes of the Spanish painter Zurburan and his still lifes, where the operative word is 'still'. Each pot, each plate, each book or loaf of bread or woven basket, has 'a heightened presence', and partly due to how the artist places them in relation to each other, and partly due to the fall of light which gives them a strange luminosity, 'these ordinary material things feel mystical, luminous, holy'. They are 'imbued with a sacramental feeling. Everything feels *seen*.'[20]

Towards the end of *King Lear*, the blinded Gloucester meets Lear on the cliffs near Dover. Lear asks him: 'yet you see how this world goes?' and Gloucester replies: 'I see it *feelingly*.'[21] To see things 'feelingly', with insight, is to respect the creation, to accept that we have 'a responsibility to awe'. I think of Blake's words: 'I sometimes look at a knot in a piece of wood until I am frightened at it' ('frightened' in the sense of 'awestruck'); and 'If the doors of perception were cleansed everything would appear as it is, infinite.' Ruskin, setting up his Working Men's College in the East End of London, urges his students to learn to draw so that they may come to see each thing in its 'thisness', what Hopkins called its 'inscape', its inner integrity, and Ruskin's own drawings of a feather, a crab, a stone, capture the absolute distillation of featherness, crabbiness and stoniness. Ted Hughes explains how he seeks in his poetry to capture the essence of a bird or an animal, of how, in an act of imaginative empathy, he seeks 'to imagine it, see it, look at it, touch it, smell it, listen to it, turn yourself into it ...' And Rilke (as I wrote earlier), with his passionate belief that the holy is to be found in the ordinary, writes that the creation may be redeemed bit by bit by an act of transforming attention, for that is to name it with what amounts to an act of love.

... and reflecting on Jesus (1)

In today's *Church Times* Giles Fraser writes of how we inevitably create our own image of God, and need to distrust it, as it says so much more about us than about God. We think of Jesus as our own 'type' (to use Myers Briggs language). The introvert will think of him as an introvert, the extrovert as an extrovert. True enough, up to a point. We see Jesus as we want to see him. All my ministry I have taken the 'soft' approach, played down sin and judgement (so dominant in the Middle Ages and in present-day fundamentalism), played up mercy and compassion, seen the essence of Jesus' ministry as affirming individuals, not excluding them, seen the Kingdom as elusive and full of surprises. Ironically, when I retired from the Abbey, one of my gifts was an icon, painted by Sergei Fedorov, the young Russian icon-maker who produced the fine icons we commissioned which so transformed the Abbey nave. When my icon arrived it was a stern, unsmiling Christ in dark colours, his eyes fixed on a point somewhere above my head. I suspect I needed that bit of balance and soon grew to value it, even if at times like the present I yearn for a more tender gaze. (Perhaps that's my strange, fatherless, rather lonely childhood speaking.) For I realise that my icon suggests the Gethsemane Christ, the one who shares the suffering. That's the Christ I need now. One who, being human, was tempted in that garden to turn back from the inevitable outcome, but held true to his vocation.

Many would write off the whole religious story and the search for God as no more than a childish need for comfort and assurance projected onto a transcendent, supernatural being who simply doesn't exist. Yet it's just as valid to see the human sense of incompleteness, the reaching out for God, as the truest and deepest and most intuitive sense of what it means to be human, one created in the likeness of the true ground and source of all that exists. Atheists make a powerful case – not least against the intransigence of those who refuse to interpret the Scriptures with any critical sense – but it becomes a series of cheap jibes when it ignores the great weight of evidence for believing that the whole creation is permeated by Mind, and is content merely to rubbish the easiest targets, those extremists who are wholly unrepresentative of generations of thoughtful believers.

Such a condescending dismissal of what so many hold important is irritating. For it's merely perverse not to recognise as valid a universal and continuing quest for the Other, a desire of the human spirit to explore that which lies just out of reach. Of course there are many misinterpretations of the demands of religious faith. There have always been and no doubt always will be many terrible and inhumane things done in Christ's name (and Muhammad's); as many images of the unimaginable source of our lives whom we call 'God' and of Jesus as there are human beings, some more dotty than others, and all of them incomplete. A thousand years ago St Bernard asked 'What is God?' and answered, 'I can think of no better answer than He who is.' And in one of his *Sermons on the Song of Songs* he writes:

> I have gone up to the highest that I have, and behold, the Word was towering yet higher. My curiosity took me to the lowest depths to look for Him, nevertheless He was found still deeper.

If I looked outside me, I found He was beyond my farthest; if I looked within he was more inward still.

The witness of the world faith communities may sometimes seem puzzlingly diverse, but their robust testimony to the character of ultimate reality can't just be written off. There is the experience of the mystics of the great Abrahamic faiths of Judaism, Christianity and Islam, who perceive a fusion of the One in the All, the All in the One; who see a hidden meaning and significance lying behind the phenomena of creation, and an underlying love upholding and infiltrating all that is. There is the intellect and reasoned faith of the Church Fathers, scholars and saints down the ages: Augustine and Benedict and Francis, Anselm and Bernard of Clairvaux, Julian of Norwich and Martin Luther, George Herbert and Thomas Traherne, Richard Hooker and William Law, Charles Gore and F. D. Maurice, Simone Weil and William Temple, Michael Ramsey and Rowan Williams. Mix in the splendour of Durham Cathedral; the music of Bach's Passions and Cantatas and Beethoven's *Missa Solemnis*; the art of Michelangelo, Giotto and Raphael; the founding of hospitals, schools and hospices; a history of Western civilisation and culture shot through with the most potent images of love and suffering, forgiveness and new life, stemming from the actions of Jesus of Nazareth; and the repeated story of generations of people discovering hope, comfort and courage as they struggle to make sense of suffering, many of them ready to die to defend the faith that has sustained them and given meaning to their lives. To dismiss all this as what Carlyle called 'transcendendal moonshine' is to trivialise the past and write off the integrity of millions.

Yet it would be wrong glibly to dismiss those who reject the notion of God, especially those who have been bruised – even broken – by life, who see it not as a rich privilege, but rather, in Hobbes' words, as 'solitary, poor, nasty, brutish and short'. However persuaded Christians may be of the truth of their faith, when disaster strikes, when poverty or

AIDS have you in their relentless grip, then going round (in the Psalmist's words) 'grinning like a dog' or believing in the ever-protective – and therefore selective – hand of God is to show scant regard for either life or God. 'If way to the Better there is', wrote Thomas Hardy, 'it exacts a full look at the Worst.'[22] The tragic makes no sense unless we treat life with the absolute seriousness it demands. A seriousness which is what alone gives meaning to trust and distinguishes hope from false optimism. Job's afflictions lie at the very heart of the human story, and there are no easy answers. I'm back with the Gethsemane Jesus: with a man who lived life as he wanted to live it, who on the Cross knew the passing anguish of a seeming desertion ('My God, my God, *why* ...'). We ask 'Why should men suffer? Why does evil exist?' Jesus, of all men, surely knew the force of those most human of questions; he would have studied the book of Job; he was faced endlessly with damaged, broken people who desired healing. Yet ultimately he did not question the good purpose of God. He felt the full force of the questions, but they were contained within his overriding concept of the fatherly love of the Father. Edwin Muir, in his autobiography, wrote: 'The existence of evil remains a mystery to me: I prefer that mystery to any explanation of it that I know.'[23] Jesus knew that mystery, but he was all the more concerned to proclaim the mystery of love. That, too, can't be explained, only experienced.

Must return to this, but not today. Wish I could get to my computer, but it's up a dozen steep stairs ... Tonight a huge Samuel Palmer moon comes and goes between scudding clouds, making them translucent.

20th August
Psalm at morning prayer, 42:

> Why are you so full of heaviness, O my soul,
> and why are you so disquieted within me?

O put your trust in God;
for I will yet give him thanks, who is the help of my
countenance, and my God.

Reflecting on Jesus (2)

There's more to say about our different concepts of Jesus and how we can ever know his true face. Which parts of the sometimes conflicting accounts of his words and actions in the Gospels can we accept without question, as authentic in the *now* as it was in the *then*? In the words Jesus addresses to his disciples, and by implication to us: 'Who do you say that I am?'

In Vikram Seth's book he explores the characters of his Uncle Shanti and Aunty Henny. The latter escaped from Nazi Germany in 1938 while her mother and sister died respectively in the camp of Theresienstadt and the gas-ovens of Auschwitz. He learns, with the late discovery of a trunk-load of letters, facts about both of them of which neither – though he thought he knew them well – had ever spoken, including aspects of their characters which surprised and at times shocked him; facts which it seems Shanti and Henny, although married for over 30 years, never discussed. Biographers seek to capture a person in all their different roles and penetrate behind the protective masks: parent, lover, public person, private self, knowing that not even those who share our lives and love us most know the full secrets of any human heart.

In the case of Jesus of Nazareth, the four Gospels are not seeking to be biographies. The materials for a biography are simply not there. Nor do they stand alone. Paul teases out the new post-Easter significance of the Christ, the human image of God, whereas the Gospels – even though written in the light of Easter – focus on the Jesus of history. Paul knows that the young churches' experience of Jesus means that he must now be understood as a dynamic presence, able to enter as powerfully and challengingly as he ever did, into their lives. The four Gospels, in focusing on just three years

101

of Jesus' public ministry, and majoring on his Passion and death, are the product of those who, after many years of an oral tradition in which the account of his words and actions, and the stories he told, are endlessly repeated, know that there is a need for written scrolls which can be circulated to the rapidly growing groups of Christians and explain the grounds for their faith.

Each one is different, allowing for a diversity of pictures of Jesus which will appeal to people according to their background and temperament, but giving scope for later biblical literalists to play havoc with them. There is the logic and order of the somewhat legalistic Matthew, the more graphic narrative style of Mark, the strong emphasis in Luke on the humanity of Jesus, with his compassionate inclusion of the oppressed and the lost, and the mystical approach of the more intuitive John, who has meditated for a lifetime on the significance of this charismatic man, and declares him at the start to be the Logos, the Word, the creative power of God, made flesh. John plucks Jesus from his Jewish background and universalises him, using words that will be understood and win a response in the Greek-speaking world into which the faith is now spreading. He speaks of Jesus as the one 'closest to the Father's heart' and many believe that what is almost certainly the last of the Gospels to be included in the canon comes closest to the heart of Jesus. For John, as for Paul, the emphasis is on the paradox of Jesus' humanity and divinity, which had gradually become the central tenet of Christian belief because of the undeniable experience of those who had known him. They didn't question that he was fully and painfully human. But equally there was no doubt that in him lay the power to heal and transform their lives. Or that this life-giving power was of God. This was an experience for which the words had not yet been invented, and even after two millennia we can only (in Emily Dickinson's words) 'tell it slant'.

How can I know that emerging from these diverse literary portraits I can discover the authentic Jesus, the one whose authority still makes a claim on my life; the one who can transform my life, so that (in Paul's phrase) 'if anyone is in Christ, he is a new creature'? By discerning the truths that run like golden threads through this heady mix of miracles, parables, promises, threats, exhortations, and words of both challenge and comfort: his overwhelming sense of the Father's presence pervading all things; his passionate concern for truth and for the poor and the oppressed. What I have earlier called the *cantus firmus* of his teaching and self-sacrifice and therefore of my faith: the enduring melody of the Kingdom. The implications of the Kingship of Christ. What Jesus calls us to discover is what Hugh (in a lovely phrase) calls 'the Kingdom-heart'. If you have it, then all else follows: a new way of seeing God and his justice and compassion, both equally demanding; the breadth of his welcome, the tender concern that nevertheless leaves us free, the unobtrusive hidden presence that to us inevitably *feels* like absence. It isn't simply learning to see God with new eyes, but learning to see people and things as God sees them, to see them for what they are: each one unique and of infinite worth.

For the early Christians to know that Jesus was alive was not to sit around puzzling about the mystery of the Easter appearance, but to see all people with love and the world lit with hope. This is what he had taught them. Not just the truth about God, but the truth of what it is to be fully and truly human. Of course we are face-to-face with mystery. But need we complicate things quite as much as some theologians seem to do? There was a piece of graffiti in an American university which read:

> Jesus said to them, 'Who do you say that I am?' And they replied, 'You are the eschatological manifestation of the ground of our being, the kerygma of which we find the ultimate meaning in our interpersonal relationships.' And Jesus said, 'What?'

Theologians have usually begun with God and what it means for Jesus to be called 'the Son of God' who came to reveal the Father, and then drawn up credal statements which have sometimes united Christians, but just as often divided them. What may be more fruitful is to begin with man, to see Jesus as a mirror in which we may see our humanity. 'Man', said Karl Barth, 'is the creature made visible in the mirror of Jesus Christ.' Words echoed by the Orthodox priest and teacher, Fr Dimitriu Stanisloe, who wrote: 'The glory to which humanity is called is that we should grow more and more God-like by becoming more and more human.' And by St Augustine, who said: 'Make humanity your way and you shall arrive at God.' As the author of the fourteenth-century English spiritual classic *The Cloud of Unknowing* put it: 'To our intellect God is evermore incomprehensible.' But not to our love: 'By love he may be gotten and holden: by thought never.' And Jesus, in both defining and living out what love is and how love acts, invites us to discover our true potential and, in so doing, discover God. So the only place to begin is where Jesus' first disciples began: with this man who leads us to a deeper understanding of human life and of God as their Father. Would we have loved/admired/been attracted to him *as a man*? Then that's where we start now, and if we can make the shift between 'then' and 'now' it is because of the mystery of the resurrection and the giving of the Spirit.

A 'responsibility to awe'. There is a kind of 'my-pal-Jesus' familiarity that is in danger of keeping him firmly trapped in the role of the charismatic carpenter of Nazareth, and where all sense of mystery vanishes. (A radio evangelist in the United States, George Vaudeman, combining those two traditional American obsessions, religion and food, was advising listeners on 'what to offer Jesus if he paid a visit to your house. I'm sure a peanut-butter-and-jelly sandwich would be fine with him,' the pastor said, 'but when you make that sandwich for Jesus, be sure you make it with wholemeal bread.') For the humanity is not where it ended for the first disciples. By the time Paul is writing, the Jesus many had known in the flesh had become the 'image of the invisible God': the authentic icon of the eternally Christlike God. Their worship was 'through Jesus Christ our Lord' as they asked that their hopes and desires, and their whole response to life, might be fashioned by the love he disclosed. It isn't a question of leaving behind the Jesus of the Gospel-writers, or making a clear distinction between the Jesus of history and the Christ of faith, but of embracing this unique human being who disclosed the full significance of *human* only when it comes to reflect the image of the divine. To know (not just to know about) Jesus in this profound sense may lead to us assenting to many of the central doctrines of incarnation and redemption if we come to understand them in ways that meet the tests of reason and conscience. It will also lead to a fresh desire to worship God with the new insight Jesus gives into his nature; and, in the light of his teaching about love of neighbour which derives from the truth of the universal love of God for all, to do so with others in word and sacrament within the gathered community of the Church.

Watched impressive televised performance of Beethoven's *Choral Symphony* from the Proms.

21st August

Get to the cathedral Eucharist, albeit in a wheelchair. My father took his life in 1933 and I only have two of his possessions: a pair of ivory-backed hairbrushes with most of the bristles missing, and a large, frayed Paisley silk square which I have not worn since my Cambridge thespian under-graduate days 50 years ago, when cravats, coloured waistcoats and thick tweed jackets were *de rigueur*. How absurd we were! Don it this morning to disguise my scarred and swollen neck. Can now descend the 13 stairs to our basement dining-room and the 13 stairs to the bedroom without stopping a few times *en route*.

As I write, a large, very handsome, bottle-green Emperor dragonfly is perched on the drainpipe three feet away. Such tiny things help to lighten the day. In her recent book of prose essays, *Findings*,[24] the Scottish poet Kathleen Jamie observes with delight the small wonders of nature as she travels from her home in Fife to Aberdeen and Orkney, the Hebrides and the central Highlands. She watches the shore birds rising together and banking 'like when you pull the string of a Venetian blind', the solitary falcon shrieking 'thinly over and over, like a turnstile pleading for oil'. She keeps on her desk the delicate skull of a gannet. But the darkness is never far away. Her mother suffers a stroke, her grandmother must be eased gently into residential care, her husband is rushed to hospital with a life-threatening disease of the blood. And she copes, not by turning to a God in whom she does not believe, but by concentrating on such tiny natural wonders as a spider's web, the carcass of a starling, the look of a patient's foot, the body-language of the doctor. And she wonders if this giving proper attention may be a form of secular prayer, 'the care and maintenance of our noticing, the paying heed'. Which brings to mind Carol Ann Duffy's small poem, 'Prayer', about the continuing need, where orthodox beliefs and approaches to prayer have fallen out of fashion, to fall back on what Jamie calls 'secular prayer' to fill the gap:

> Some days, although we cannot pray, a prayer
> utters itself. So, a woman will lift
> her head from the sieve of her hands and stare
> at the minims sung by a tree, a sudden gift ...
>
> Pray for us now. Grade I piano scales
> console the lodger looking out across
> a Midlands town. Then dusk, and someone calls
> a child's name as though they named their loss ...
>
> Darkness outside. Inside, the radio's prayer –
> Rockall. Malin. Dogger. Finisterre.[25]

Tonight's bit of nostalgia is *Casablanca*. What a cast! What a film!

22nd August

Morning prayer Psalm 119:37: 'Turn my eyes from watching what is worthless': *Celebrity Big Brother* certainly: surely not *Casablanca*? Card from publishers commissioning this book unseen and offering a contract. I ask them to put it on hold. Let's just see what the next months may bring.

Reflecting on words (1)

I've been thinking about words, both their power and their inadequacy to define the commonest things – a ray of light, say, or the colour blue. How to describe human consciousness and the mystery of the 'self' or the mystic's experience of God? 'Hints and guesses' said Eliot, and how dull life would be if the scientists could write 'QED' under all the questions about *how* the world works, and all the philosophers and theologians could give neat answers to the '*why?*' questions about the meaning of our existence. Silence is often the only option. As St Francis is alleged to have said, when sending out his followers to preach the Gospel: 'Use words, too, if you must.' Those ascetic fourth-century monks in the deserts of Egypt, Syria and Palestine whom we call the Desert Fathers spent their time wrapped in an almost unimaginable depth of inner silence. They taught by simply 'being', not by speech. One wrote, 'If a man cannot understand my silence, he will never understand my words.' At a less exalted level, it's said that Einstein was a very late starter when it came to speaking, and that his first words were, 'This milk is too hot.' When asked why he hadn't spoken previously, he replied, 'Because everything was in order.'

Language was the most vital breakthrough in the long climb from the stardust that became the primordial soup; from the first green plants and primitive cells with their self-producing molecules; from the invertebrates, the fish, the amphibians, the reptiles and the mammals – a time when dragonflies as big as ravens flew among giant, moss-covered trees – to the primates; and a million years ago (after some 4000 million years of patient evolution) the emergence of *homo erectus*, the first human being. Did the apes have a kind of language? Perhaps. Experiments with sign language have shown that apes can respond to words, but haven't a hope of stringing them together. When we began to use words, perhaps some 50,000 years ago, our brains took their most significant evolutionary leap. And in due course writers were committing to paper, in story or myth, verse or prose, descriptions of what it felt like to be alive, and recording their experience of love and pain, peace and war, life and death, in terms which make the best of them as relevant to our computer age as to the Elizabethans or the ancient Greeks. Seamus Heaney speaks of writers who can lift the reader's hand and 'put it on the bare wire of the present': an image, a phrase, an idea, that strikes us as true, even universal. No matter when or where a writer lived his or her life, he or she may tell you something you need to know about your own. Even something you have in a sense always known, but never absorbed until now. In Alan Bennett's fine play, *The History Boys*, the unorthodox English teacher, Hector, passionate about education but scathing of exams, says of one of Hardy's poems:

> The best moments in reading are when you come across something – a thought, a feeling, a way of looking at things – which you had thought special and peculiar to you. Now here it is, set down by someone else, a person you have never met, someone even who is long dead. And it is as if a hand has come out and taken yours.[26]

Language seeks to define and pin down our shared experiences and discoveries, but ultimately has to admit to only partial triumphs, and must make way for other forms of communication: music and art and dance, listening and silence. Sally Purcell, a poet who died in her fifties in 1998, writes in 'Poem for Lent or Advent':

> Signs and shadows
> have been gathering reality

as they rush upward
to the surface of time;
they break
into our mind's air, snatch us through
knowledge of the visible,

through the game of images,
into that Love
who sawed both cross and cradle
out of the same tree.[27]

It is the 'signs and shadows' of a different reality at work in what we call Incarnation, Cross and Resurrection, that take us through 'knowledge of the visible' and 'the game of images' into a true discovery of that Love which, in the words of Dante, 'moves the sun and the other stars', and which poets as well as theologians seek, and inevitably fail, to capture in mere words. Ultimately God addresses us in the only terms which we can understand, when in the incomparable words of the Fourth Gospel, 'the Word was made flesh and dwelt among us, full of grace and truth'. In Genesis we read that it is by his Word that God creates the heavens and the earth: here is its echo and fulfilment. The Word understood as the creative power of God who, in the myth that Darwin challenged but didn't destroy (for it contains a valid and equally powerful kind of truth), observes his creation as it comes into being (over all those unimaginable millennia) and finds it 'very good'.

For as long as we have had language God has been addressed in a thousand different tongues. But God speaks none of them. Or should that be 'all of them'? For God hears only the music of the heart with all its desires and longings, hopes and fears, and moments of gratitude, shame, stillness and wonder. 'The Word ... made flesh': no definition quite suffices. The word is something of yourself that you offer to another, something (at its best and most authentic) which comes from the heart and speaks of who you truly are, so that over the years it helps define your unique integrity. But

109

applied to the unknowable God? Gregory Palamas, one of the wisest of Orthodox theologians, said seven centuries ago that in all statements about God there must always be paradox and silence. Yet even the description of God as 'wholly Other', indicating his absolute difference from his creation, has to be held in a fine balance by the truth that we can only begin to meet this 'otherness' by dint of the fact that he has made himself known to us in the midst of history, in that crucial moment of the Incarnation. 'The Word ... made flesh', and so not quite unknowable: the boy who could be reprimanded by Mary and Joseph (as in Simone Martini's marvellous painting in Liverpool's Walker Art Gallery, where a defiant 12-year-old stands stubborn and unmoved in the face of his parents' bewilderment); the Jewish rabbi who spoke words that took fire in the hearts of some who heard them, and caused anger when they cut through the engrained legalistic claims of the orthodox; the flesh that was tortured and nailed up to die between two thieves. Yes, we can understand 'flesh'. It's vulnerable and easily destroyed. But what of 'full of grace and truth'? Well, that's what this journal is seeking to rediscover, and no dictionary definitions will do. But that's enough for one day.

As I'm listening in bed to Mozart's *Requiem*, Frederick Buechner phones from Vermont. He is a greatly valued friend. Hugely popular in the States for his novels, auto-biographical writing and sermons full of humane theology, he is hardly published in Britain. Those who don't know his work should log on to Amazon and try for starters *The Alphabet of Grace*, *Telling the Truth*, or *Godric*.

23rd August

A cloudless morning. Writing from Yorkshire, where they are filming *The History Boys*, Alan B. tells me how, after his major operation for cancer, he used 'to look forward to *anything* – valium, morphine, pre-med. – just because it made a change from boring old me'. A. drives me up to Old

110

Sarum. Walk, at a geriatric pace, some 200 yards. Couldn't have done that a week ago.

Reflecting on words (2)

Watching the finches squabbling on the bird-feeder, I'm still thinking about what Eliot in 'Little Gidding' calls 'the intolerable wrestle/ With words and meanings'; of how ('East Coker') they 'crack and sometimes break, under the burden/ Under the tension, slip, slide, perish,/ Decay with imprecision .../ Will not stay still'. And theological words are sometimes the ones that are most liable to cracking and breaking, decaying with imprecision as each generation fingers them afresh, holds them up to the light, and asks if they are still valid in the context of new ways of understanding the universe and human consciousness, questions of gender and what makes us who we are; and the nature of society as it too slips and slides and (to the despair of the elderly and the traditionalists) will not stay in place.

John Wesley says that preachers should 'constantly use the common, little, easy words ... which our language affords'. Yet the simple may too easily become the simplistic. And we should look to the professional wordsmiths – the poets, novelists and playwrights – as they seek to shift, however imperceptibly, the way we perceive the world. The poet Don Paterson believes that all good poets walk the tightrope between sense and mystery, making sense but pointing to the mystery.

> The universe our senses conjure up for us is not the universe. We know that the ears of the bat, the eyes of the bee, the nose of the dog, the sensitivity of the bird to magnetic field ... shape a perception of the world wholly different from our own, yet no more or less true.[28]

Those who seek to preach or write about their faith are, in Paul's words, 'stewards of the *mysteries*': we need, like Lear, to 'take upon's the mystery of things'. The best users of words know that truth is an evasive mistress, and that images, metaphors, stories, myth, have a better hope of netting at least some aspects of the mystery that lies all about and within us. The writer Hilary Mantel, reviewing a recent novel, writes of it as 'austere, authoritative fiction, a fine melancholy novel, its poignant insights shimmering, just as they should do, a little space beyond the powers of summary or analysis'.[29] Exactly. That very fine contemporary poet, John Burnside, knows that the more we know about anything (or anyone), the more the mystery deepens; that the whole is always greater than the sum of the parts. He captures the sense of the interdependence of all living things, the paradox of time and the moments which seem to intrude on eternity; the distinction between what we *know* and what we *are*; and the relationship between human beings and nature. He seeks to name the unnameable, as in his poem 'Kith':

> ... what we know is mostly the agreed
> and measured, what we are is something else
>
> and never comes
> without some inattention:
> light on a kitchen wall, light on a face,
>
> a truth that resides
> in the details: the ebb and flow
>
> of seasons
> and the world we paraphrase
> as crease and furrow; grass-blade; robin's nest;
>
> the *terra incognita* of the whole.[30]

What artists and writers attempt to do, in paint or words, is to capture the transient moment, to trap our fleeting vision and passing sensation before the memory fades, to show us what has mattered to them and what we may have missed. In her book on fundamentalism in Judaism, Christianity and Islam,[31] Karen Armstrong clarifies the difference

112

between *myth* and *logos*. According to Plato, there are two complementary ways of arriving at truth, both of equal weight. *Logos* (reason) is the rational, the scientific, spelled out in facts which are capable of logical explanation and in words which are unsubtle and easily comprehended. Myth, on the other hand, deals with *meaning*, with stories which help to convey what is timeless and unchanging. It relates to the intuitive and is best expressed in art, music or ritual. She explains how they clarify different aspects of the world, but that as a result of the scientific revolution, where *logos* triumphed so spectacularly that myth was discredited, 'people in the western world began to think that *logos* was the only means to truth, and began to discount *mythos* as false and superstitious ... and read the biblical myths as though they were *logoi*'. To confuse these two necessary ways of apprehending the reality of the world leads to creationism, to the fundamentalists' attempt to read the Bible (or the Koran) in a literal way that would not have made sense in an earlier age. Fundamentalism, writes George Steiner, 'is that blind lunge towards simplification, and the infantile comforts of imposed discipline'.[32] Words can be dangerous weapons when they are waved around without much understanding of the subtle, complex nature of truth.

The Bible records the centuries-long exploration into what the nature of God may be, and why we are here. The culmination (for Christians) of this journey by the people of Israel, with all its false turnings and dead ends, bloody wars and sudden shafts of insight, is the young Jewish rabbi who was strung up on a gibbet on a Friday and who was believed to have been raised by God three days later. Christian dogmas are subsequent attempts to discern the truth lurking behind the familiar stories. For they are clearly undeniable for those who knew him and who claim:

> It was there from the beginning; we have heard it; we have seen it with our own eyes; we looked upon it, and felt it with our own hands; our theme is the Word which gives life. This life

was made visible ... we declare to you the eternal life which was with the Father and was made visible to us.[33]

In the New Testament this message is often woven with mythical elements, for the Gospels were written for people for whom it was natural to think mythologically, to discern the truth through stories. New truths and experiences of faith were (are) often best conveyed in this way. The stories of a birth in a stable, or an empty tomb in a garden, are far more powerful images to manifest faith than a wordy attempt to define divine sonship or the meaning of resurrection. We need stories as much as ever: whether it is Wagner's *Ring* cycle or Tolkein's *Lord of the Rings*, C. S. Lewis's *Narnia*, Harry Potter or Philip Pullman's *Dark Materials* trilogy, all contain tested truths about the nature of the battle between good and evil. The question is: which are the myths of the Bible which are simply made up stories to illustrate general truths, and which are events told in myth form *because that is the best (sometimes the only) way their truth may be discerned*? For, while the claims of the Christian faith are based on historical events, their meaning often lies just beyond the power of plain words to convey.

Many of the biblical myths and images need to be distinguished from historical accounts and understood for what they are: memorable stories conveying a truth. We need to sort the *mythos* from the *logos*. Jesus knew that truth is not always best conveyed by reciting the unadorned facts, that just as there are different forms of reality, so there are different forms of truth. A man attacked by robbers on the way from Jerusalem to Jericho might earn a short paragraph in the local paper; a dissolute son returning home to his family might be of passing interest in the village; but what have they to do with us? The story of the Good Samaritan or the Prodigal Son, however, speak powerfully of my relationship with God, and the nature of compassion and forgiveness; truths which touch me deeply and will be as relevant for our children's children as they were for their first hearers. As Hans Kung has written: 'The Bible is interested primarily not in historical truth, but in truth relevant for our well-being, for our salvation.'

'Primarily', note, for unless its stories arose out of certain historical facts it would just be a story book. It's easy enough to get the point of the creation-myth of Eden, and those of the Flood or the parting of the Red Sea, but when it comes to the New Testament, what do we make of the stories of the virgin birth, the miracles of Jesus, or the Resurrection? We shall never know what really happened, but the question is what these stories *mean for us*. Like Italo Calvino's definition of a classic, the New Testament 'has never finished saying what it has to say'. This is tricky ground, calling for a book rather than a few jottings by a convalescent in a journal. But briefly:

(i) We know rather less about the events of Jesus' birth, ministry, death and raising to new life than the powerful effect they had on the subsequent Christian community.

(ii) The four Gospels adopt differing styles in order to set out their life-changing truths in the most powerful and appealing way they can, but do so several decades after the events and in the transforming light of Easter. So, while some of the 'miracle' stories (walking on the water, the multiplication of loaves and fishes, the raising of Lazarus) go against the laws of nature, they convey the truth in story form of what they now see God has done through Jesus to display the healing, sharing, life-giving and death-defeating signs of the new order he has initiated, the Kingdom.

(iii) The stories of the shepherds, the star and the birth in a stable are perhaps introduced by Matthew and Luke to reflect the naked vulnerability of the one destined to confront the power of Rome with his universal message of the seeming powerlessness (yet deceptive power) of self-giving love; the one whose first concern is with the poor and the marginalised. The Saviour not just of Israel but (hence the story of the Magi) of all humankind.

(iv) The idea of a virgin birth was a widespread myth in

the religions of the ancient world and not specifically Christian. The story of the birth of Jesus seems to have been unknown to Paul and isn't mentioned by Mark or John. Here again, myth meets *logos*: a human birth set in a story which provides a framework for theological reflection; what Paul came to understand as the divine sonship, 'God in Christ reconciling the world to himself', and what John came to call 'the Word made flesh'. Yet to us, knowing the biological fact that to be a human being you need 23 pairs of chromosomes, and in each pair one from the father and one from the mother, it appears to challenge Jesus' authentic humanity. However, the idea of the virgin birth has proved an enduring and meaningful symbol of the truth that in Jesus there is a new creation. As long ago as 1922, in the Doctrine Report chaired by Archbishop William Temple, they wrote:

> It is a safeguard of the Christian conviction that in the Person of Christ humanity made a fresh beginning ... There are, however, some among us who hold ... that belief in the historical Incarnation is more consistent with the supposition that our Lord's birth took place under the normal conditions of human generation. In their minds the notion of a Virgin Birth tends to mar the completeness of the belief that in the Incarnation God revealed Himself at every point in and through human nature.[34]

(v) The empty tomb; the meeting with Mary Magdalen in the garden; the upper room and the story of Thomas; the breakfast at the lakeside; the walk to Emmaus where he was known in the breaking of bread. These are memorable, persuasive stories, perhaps even more so for their lack of harmony in trying to describe the indescribable. They're written to help explain the triumphant emergence of groups of people ready to suffer and die for their belief that 'Jesus is Lord' after the finality of Good Friday. None claim to have witnessed the actual Resurrection: what those who figure in these stories claim is to have encountered the living Jesus, raised by God from death. The story of Jesus is all of a piece, a revolutionary event, something utterly new, which is why history now tips over from BC to AD. Resurrection, like the original act of creation, is not against the laws of nature. It is a new act of God, 'the One who calls into existence the things that are not',[35] and is now seen to be able to call the unique identity who was Jesus (and therefore, by implication, the unique identity who is me) out of death into new, unimaginable life. Faith in the Resurrection is inseparable from faith in God. If we question it, maybe that is because our concept of God is so inadequate.

The Scottish theologian T. F. Torrance imagines a reporter trying to find the words which will make sense of these events in the light of the Resurrection:

> Then gradually as the material takes shape under his pen in a remarkable inherence of words and events, he is aware that under the creative impact of the resurrection something like a new literary form is struggling to come into being. His reporting has to take on a new character to do justice to its subject-matter; and yet that is precisely what it cannot really do: it has to be shaped in such a way that it indicates and bears witness to more than it can formally express.[36]

How, then, shall we describe this God of a hundred names? The German Jesuit Karl Rahner wrote this prayer:

> What can I say to you, my God? Shall I collect together all the words that praise your holy name? Shall I give you all the names of this world, you, the Unnameable? Shall I call you 'God of my life, meaning of my existence, hallowing of my acts, my journey's end, bitterness of my bitter hours, home of my loneliness, you my most treasured happiness'? Shall I say: Creator, Sustainer, Pardoner, Near One, Distant One, Incomprehensible One, God both of flowers and stars, God of the gentle wind and of terrible battles, Wisdom, Power, Loyalty and Truthfulness, Eternity and Infinity, you the All-Merciful, you the Just One, you Love itself?

How shall we describe God? In so many different ways, but 'He who raised Jesus from the dead' has to be among them.

24th August: Reflecting on God (3)

Words from this morning's Psalm, 145: 'The Lord is loving to everyone and his compassion is over all his works', echoed by some words of Anselm set as a canticle:

> Lord Jesus, in your mercy heal us;
> in your love and tenderness, remake us.
> In your compassion, bring grace and forgiveness;
> for the beauty of heaven, may your love prepare us ...

make me reflect that the Psalmist had no doubts (nor did the major prophets, for all their fierce denunciations) that what they spoke of as God's 'wrath' is more than matched by his mercy and lovingkindness. We too feel angry at blatant injustice. But somehow this deep insight of Judaism into God's sheer grace was constantly threatened by the stranglehold of the legalistic mind, the Pharasaic desire to enforce a moral code which was never very tender and rarely compassionate, and in so doing drain the life of the spirit out of religious practice. (And how often subsequently has the Church twisted Jesus' liberating concept of the Kingdom into a series of moral injunctions and an unattractive obsession with the rules.) What Jesus does as a good rabbi is to honour the law and the Mosaic code, but strip away those deadly accretions, that dry legalism, and point people back to the reality of a loving, forgiving, gracious Source, a hidden, inviting Presence whom, he told them, was best addressed as 'Father'.

'Father'. It's a word that needs time – perhaps a lifetime – to assimilate and truly make our own. The analogy with a human parent isn't necessarily helpful. My own father's suicide, while I think of him only with compassion, was in fact, for my mother and me, an act of betrayal, a betrayal of trust. And my mother, in her times of unhappiness and frequent search for love (she was widowed three times) often made emotional demands of me which could paralyse my own emotions and inhibit my response. Rainer Maria Rilke, when he interprets the parable of the Prodigal Son, can't help relating it to his own life (in which for the first few years his mother had dressed him in girl's clothes, treating him as a longed-for daughter), and sees the younger son leaving home 'for a far country' as his need to escape a suffocating love. Love which is a parody of the true thing, a clinging, demanding emotion rather than a true giving of oneself for the sake of the loved one. 'He did not want', writes Rilke, 'to be loved like this.' (Samuel Beckett was to write to his dominating mother, accusing her of loving him 'with a savage loving', fluctuating all his life between compassion and irritation, attendance and retreat.) Yet Jesus uses that story to illustrate what for many, in the detail of the father going out to greet and embrace his returning child, is the most powerful analogy of that gracious acceptance of the ever-forgiving God: what the *Book of Common Prayer* calls his 'fatherly goodness', epitomised by the image of the father's rough hands clasping his son's back, which forms the pivotal point in Rembrandt's great picture. And time and again the grace of God is reflected in Jesus as his words are 'made flesh' and take root in individual lives – Peter, Zacchaeus, Mary Magdalen, the woman taken in adultery – as they find echoed in him that same unconditional embrace.

All of us fail at times to meet this ideal. Even the best parents can sometimes let down their children, and children betray their parents. Which is why mutual forgiveness must always be a fallback factor in every loving relationship. Yet it is this loyalty, this instinctive, protective love which can be our greatest gift to our children (and perhaps, a little later in life, our greatest gift to our parents). Those lucky enough to have known what a parent's love can be are able to prosper from that experience; others, less fortunate, may nevertheless find that same quality of loyalty in the life commitment that marriage or partnership entails, or in friendship. What those things teach us about the meaning of an unchanging and constant loyalty and trust is an indication of what 'Father' hints at when applied to God. It becomes a kind of shorthand for what it means to be held by One who is 'closer to us than breathing, nearer than hands and feet', even in those dispiriting moments when we feel empty or tested beyond what seems bearable.

The Lord's Prayer ends with the seemingly strange phrase, 'lead us not into temptation' (or 'do not put us to the test'), 'but deliver us from evil' (that which will harm us). I see this cancer as putting me to 'the test', if only a modest one compared with the much more forbidding tests people face daily: an inoperable tumour (*later*: little did I know), the slow descent of someone greatly loved into Alzheimer's, the battle with black depression, the death of a child. The sudden accident or illness which (in the words of A. S. Byatt, who lost her son in a cycling accident) can 'scythe through the fabric of dailiness, and change things for ever'. Only those who endure such things know how it challenges them, and if and how they are tempted to deny whatever faith they may have in a loving God as they batter heaven with the Job-like 'Why me? Why him? Why her?' In the words of six-year-old Katie: 'Daddy's secretary was only 29 and she died in a car crash. Why wasn't God looking?' Or those of the father of an eleven-year-old son dying of leukaemia: 'Does my Creator weep?'

I've not felt the need to ask that question. However baffling they may seem at times, I can still grasp the main implications of freedom. The world is an intriguing mixture of the predetermined and the inexplicable, yet there are still sufficient determined laws of nature to allow us to speak of a dependable order in creation without which scientists would be stumbling in the dark and which point to a purposeful Mind. ('My own religious freedom,' wrote Einstein, 'takes the form of a rapturous amazement at the harmony of natural law.') Yet the human freedom to make wrong choices seems to imply a freedom in nature as well, in which order must accommodate random chance. That's the real poser, to which none of us knows the answer. In the miracle that is a human being, the trillions of atoms co-operating daily to keep us alive and healthy, there is always the risk that a foetus may abort, a baby be born disabled, cells turn cancerous. At some point, even for the healthiest, the body will wear out and die. And as Job discovered, God does not intervene. Why? Because God is not the great Puppet Master pulling the strings from somewhere out of sight. Nor is God static, for ever complete in the perfection of his creation. The Bible never conceives of him in stillness, but rather in movement, of a creation still unfinished; and the Judaeo-Christian story is so striking because it tells of a loving, suffering God working through the Jewish nation and its prophets, through Jesus and those who follow him, and through the work of the Spirit. Delivering us from evil. Inviting our freely given co-operation to win the world to himself, and establish his Kingdom where (having been tested, perhaps, almost beyond their endurance) the broken will be healed, the hungry will be fed and all will discover the home they long for.

God is like a creative artist, the Source of a universe whose laws allow the element of randomness and choice which enables its Creator to interact with a world that is an open system; one who has woven a web of life which has over billions of years evolved into those who reflect his likeness; a world of almost limitless potential for good – and therefore also for evil. If Shakespeare is a genius of the tragi-comic, that's because he succeeds in reflecting the two constants of the tragi-comic story of our days: laughter and grief, happiness and pain. To speak of God as all-powerful is confusing if that conveys a sense of one who directs and dictates our lives, and whose nature is so volatile that he creates floods and earthquakes and tumours because he is angry or displeased with us. That would make a nonsense of the core Christian belief that the most accurate definition of God is Christ crucified, the ultimate symbol of dislocation and shared vulnerability. Rather, he seems to be a Creator who, in an act of divine self-limitation, *relinquishes control over creation*, allowing it and its creatures to be self-creative as we seek for beauty and goodness and truth, and struggle to learn the meaning of the stewardship of nature, the power of reconciliation and the language of love. The result is a world in which much is allowed to happen that is far from being in accord with God's beneficent will.

Thirty years ago Rowan Williams wrote of how we must see the creation 'as that from which God withdraws to let it be itself', and God as one who in a sense 'abandons it, devoid of any unambiguous signs of his presence'. For without the spur to search for God and find meaning in our lives, and above all to protest passionately against the darkness, there would be no incentive for the finer human qualities to emerge: hope and faith and compassion. Rowan Williams writes:

> To feel and show compassion to a creature is to accept it unconditionally, and this unconditional acceptance is the action of God ... It is this compassion (in us) ... which makes God present in the world, uniting creatures to God ... The compassionate man ... directs the world towards reconciliation, brings the glory of God into the world, *even as he protests at its outrage* [my italics]. His protest witnesses to a 'possible future', the knowledge that things might be otherwise.[37]

So George Herbert, in 'The Pulley', speaks of God with-holding the gift of what he calls 'rest' from all the gifts showered on man, in order that we might be *restless* in our search for God and the things of God. Without our restless freedom to explore, without this risky choice whereby we have the potential to create or destroy, without the need to be tested in the face of the darkness of sickness and death, the Godlike gifts of altruistic love and its offshoots, for-giveness and the desire for justice, would have been still-born. Nor would there be the need for the creative arts, which not only illuminate and celebrate the human condition but so strikingly protest against the forces ranged against us. Dylan Thomas prefaces his collected poems with the words: 'These poems . . . are written for the love of Man' (i.e. feelings of compassion, anger, protest) 'and in praise of God' (the sense of hope, the awareness of grace), 'and I'd be a damn' fool if they weren't.'[38]

So I understand the phrases 'do not put us to the test' and 'deliver us from evil' as both an acceptance that testing will come, and the desire that in the face of evil we shan't be tempted to abandon what we most deeply believe about God, to question him and lose our faith; that the darkness will not overwhelm us and do us harm. Yes, I find God in the evil of my cancer. Not that he sent it, but that he is to be found in it and through it: not just in the professionalism and loving care, but as a way of teaching me something more of what Hugh would call his 'dark glory'; the opportunity to grow in faith and empathy that may emerge through suffering.

So many words: I must be feeling stronger. L. phones from the clinic to say that the MRSA is no longer active. Watch more Bogart: *The Treasure of the Sierra Madre*.

25th August
A. drives me up the Woodford Valley to sit by the Avon for coffee at The Bridge. Within five minutes the heavens open. Feel a bit washed out as well. Shouldn't have written so much in the past two days. No more writing today. Listen to Mozart and watch Fourth Test.

26th August: Reflecting on love (1), marriage and companionship
My absolute dependence on A., on her sensitivity (despite her anxiety) to my fluctuating moods during these anxious weeks, and my poor attempt to be sensitive to hers, have made me reflect on what we mean by 'one flesh'. 'And we are put on earth a little space,' wrote Blake, 'That we may

learn to bear the beams of love.'[39] What has our marriage meant to us? For 40 years we have sought to create a trusting, shared space, stemming from the public witness of our marriage vows, shaped by love and enriched by children and grandchildren. And over the years, in the give-and-take of the costly exploring of that far-reaching phrase, 'for better, for worse, in sickness and in health', there has grown up a profound mutual understanding so that each knows instinctively what the other feels or, frequently, is thinking or is about to say. Even though each of us remains a unique spirit and there continue to be those deeply private places that remain hidden, even perhaps to ourselves. Richard Hoggart, looking back on nearly 60 years of married love, compares this process of 'growing into one another, growing together like plants, intertwining without entirely interlocking, and certainly without submerging' to the violin and piano in Beethoven's *Spring Sonata*, not so much a coming together of two people as the emergence of a new unity.[40] Starting out as strangers, with no linking DNA, people can grow into the most profound intimacy and friendship, and in the act of making love (not to be confused with 'having sex'), we have produced a son and a daughter whose own DNA is a unique combination of ours, which makes them more literally 'one flesh' with each of us than we are with each other.

'Until death us do part.' If, within that closest of friendships, one should die, there is no greater anguish, no more lonely experience, than that of the one flesh being wrenched in two, with no one now to share the intimacies of your life, the private jokes and references. It's the heavy price we pay for loving, and our reason tells us that we would not have it otherwise, so that perhaps in time we may come to see that the grief we have to live with is the final, and most costly, gift we have to offer to the one who has died. But reason is not uppermost in periods of grief.

Today, very many people live in a partnership – whether heterosexual or homosexual – that is outside marriage.

Where that relationship is founded on mutual trust and the affirmation of lifelong commitment, then the new possibility of entering into a secular form of lifelong commitment in a civil partnership is surely to be welcomed rather than condemned. When two people are lucky enough to discover that degree of friendship, whether within marriage or outside it, there is not a more enviable gift. (Two of our friends, entering recently into such a formal partnership and the ceremony complete, the registrar said she hoped they'd be very happy together. 'Well, we have been for the past 47 years.') Strangely, in a society obsessed with sex, friendship is not much in fashion. In the burgeoning religious communities of the twelfth century, particularly among the Cistercians, it was a hugely important topic. They saw themselves as a group of friends choosing one another in Christ, and the best known of them, who wrote on spiritual friendship, is Aelred of Rievaulx. Known as the 'Bernard of the North', Aelred was abbot at Rievaulx, an aristocrat of Anglo-Saxon descent and the first Englishman to join the order in the north of England. He argues that friendship, more than any other relationship, propels us into the heart of the divine, and remains the best analogy we have for our relationship with the one who said to his closest companions: 'There is no greater love than this, that a man should lay down his life for his friends ... And I have called you friends.'[41]

Terry Eagleton, the Oxford academic, writes of how Aristotle thought there was a way of living that enabled us to be human at its best. For him it was life according to the virtues:

> The Judaeo-Christian tradition considers that it is the life of charity or love. What this means, roughly speaking, is that we become the occasion for each other's self-realisation. It is only through being the means of your self-fulfilment that I can attain my own, and vice versa.[42]

'We become the occasion for each other's self-realisation.' In other words: those who love us make us what we are and, moreover, enable us to be fulfilled in a way that otherwise we shouldn't be. We're not loved because we are lovely: we become lovely because we are loved. Over our lives we are shaped and changed. It is through the love of our parents, partners, siblings, children, and friends and, for believers, the God hidden in that love, that we find our true self. To grow emotionally and spiritually, we need to know that we belong, first (hopefully) in the protective shell of family and then in the unprotected wider world. Our life-graph starts with the total dependence of the new-born; it passes through the stages of the growing independence of the young adult, the discovery of selfhood in leaving home and the true test of a parent's love in the letting go; and ideally, it comes to rest in a new, different kind of dependence, found in mutual relationships of love and friendship, allowing the solitary mystery that is 'me' to be modified by reaching out to the mystery that is 'you'. Where two people find that degree of trust and affirmation, together they become strong enough to meet the challenges of life and not to be overwhelmed by them, not even by the ultimate tests of sickness or old age with its inevitable reversion to a new kind of dependence. The peaks and troughs of that graph are unpredictable, but what is for sure is that we start at zero and end at zero, as the last shuddering breath leaves the body and the heart monitor levels out as horizontally as the corpse.

'We become the occasion for each other's self-realisation.' To know the affirmation of being loved (despite our faults) because we are uniquely ourselves, is the key to growing in that outward-looking love which is *agape*. Its opposite is indifference. Out of the security of the trusting, committed give-and-take of love to which both friendship and marriage witness (Rilke's love 'between two solitudes who protect and greet and touch each other') are born certain altruistic qualities of goodness and self-sacrifice, running the gamut from giving time to someone who needs attention paid to them to a life dedicated to the service of others, or even the readiness to give your life for a person or a cause. These are the human qualities that are hard to account for or explain away if there is no God in whose likeness we are created, nothing transcendent about us; if we are simply the end-product of a long evolutionary cycle marked by the survival of the fittest, and solely explicable in terms of clever cells and selfish genes.

Now it may be an obvious truth that we are a combination of what our genes have made us (nature) and what the love of others has made us (nurture), but if we are able to reach out beyond ourselves, break out of our private little boxes in openness to one another, then the obvious truth of nature-plus-nurture must be extended to embrace a new dimension, that of the transcendent. We discover what have been called 'signals of transcendence' within the bounds of our everyday experience, though they point beyond it. For example, our penchant for order, the sense that our world is ultimately ordered and trustworthy – more like Mozart than John Cage. Or in certain transparent, even timeless, moments of joy. In the persistence of hope, even in the most desperate circumstances. In our response to natural beauty and to whatever in words or art or music has proved of transcendent value to past generations. Many of these affirmations are as much Jewish and Muslim (or, indeed, human) as they are Christian.

Underlying the universal human truth that those who love us make us what we are, that we can only learn what love is by being loved, is for Christians a deeper truth. For we believe that the love which is self-giving rather than self-serving has its origin in the Mind behind the universe, which Christians claim was once expressed in history in one like us, one whose life is celebrated as the high point in the human story. John writes in his first letter, 'We love because he first loved us.' He's not saying 'we love *him*': he's saying that we human beings only have the ability to love unself-ishly (in terms of *agape*) because we have been loved into existence by God in his desire to share what lies at his heart.

Once you are persuaded that you are lovable, it changes the way you see everything: God, yourself, your neighbour. But God's love can only be mediated to us by others. We become what we first receive. That's the consistent principle. We pass on what we have been given. And those who make the leap of faith trace that love beyond its human mediators to the One we believe to be its only true (though often unacknowledged) source.

In Margaret Atwood's novel *Alias Grace*, Grace – a mid-Victorian 16-year-old serving maid – is accused of being an accomplice in the murder of her master and his butler. In prison she ponders on why she was given the name of Grace. Was she perhaps named after the hymn, 'Amazing Grace'?

> Amazing Grace, how sweet the sound,
> That saved a wretch like me!
> I once was lost, but now am found,
> Was blind but now I see.

> I hope I was named after it. I would like to be found. I would like to see. Or to be seen. I wonder if, in the eye of God, it amounts to the same thing. As it says in the Bible, *For now we see through a glass darkly; but then face to face.*
>
> If it is face to face, there must be two looking.[43]

'We become the occasion for each other's self-realisation.' An astonishing truth when related to God: we through acknowledging our relationship, God through his creation and its creatures. There's more to say, but it will have to wait till morning, as I only have the energy to return to the Fourth Test, followed by another great classic, *Cinema Paradiso*.

27th August: Reflecting on love (2)

What I wrote yesterday will have seemed impossibly idealistic: this is not life as many people know it. Many, through no fault of their own, face pretty loveless lives, ones of missing or unrequited love. Even, perhaps especially, in the rich nations of the North, the search for love proves abortive, marriages fail, divorce is at once relatively easy but emotionally costly and damaging to family life, poverty and drugs take a heavy toll. Yet a failure to live as we might doesn't invalidate the model so many achieve. Any more than those who deny the existence of God or reject concepts of him which are so warped that they are best abandoned, or who have been so hurt that they have lost whatever faith they once had, negate the validity and integrity of those who are seeking to live with 'the Kingdom-heart'. Those who persist in their commitment to relationships based on trust, mutual forgiveness and the lifelong exploration of the implications of love fail repeatedly to live up to that ideal, which is why forgiveness is part and parcel of every act of worship. Where we are often blind is in narrowing how we conceive of the love of neighbour. Teilhard de Chardin wrote that Christ's central message to the world was: 'Love one another, recognising in the heart of each of you the same God who is being born.' That implies the recognition of the common unity of all humankind, all part of what John Donne called 'the main'. Every person is made in the image of God, and Christianity becomes stiflingly insular if it is seen as primarily a means of personal salvation, rather than a way of acting together to explore the implications of the commission to exercise the love which is *agape* in both its personal and corporate manifestations.

This morning's New Testament reading was Jesus' parable of the wise and foolish bridesmaids, and how the wise refused the request of the foolish to lend them oil for their lamps when surprised by the bridegroom's sudden arrival. I understand that to mean that the qualities demanded of us in the Kingdom – a childlike trust, a concern for justice and equity, the imaginative understanding of one another's needs – can't be learned overnight or borrowed from others. This learning to trust and the discovery of what love demands, both in our closest relationships and in our wider lives, takes time, for most of us a lifetime. Nor (to return to where I started yesterday) can you begin to sense the security and liberation that a lifelong, loving commitment can bring unless you are living and growing within that confident relationship. You can test the water, as many now do, by an experimental period of living together, but that doesn't quite carry the conviction of the public declaration of vows. Equally, the only place from which to test the validity of the Christian faith is from within a Christian community. None of them may ever prove to be exactly what we desire, but it is only from within the worshipping body, centred on the word and sacraments, that we can gradually test whether the incarnate, Christlike God answers something so deep within us that it is like an unquenched thirst. Anselm's words, 'I do not seek to understand so that I may believe, but *believe that I may understand*' are sometimes mocked as being an intellectual cop-out. Yet he is merely stating what is true in every other area of our life. Doing always precedes understanding. We learn to speak before we can grasp the rules of grammar and syntax. Only when we feel a sense of the transcendent do we feel the need to explore what is meant by God. Only when we know we are loved are we set free to love. Only now, in the midst of this 'questioning country of cancer' can I speak with any real knowledge of what it feels like, and if and how God may still be found within it.

A timely card today from two Muslim friends, with two quotes from the Koran: 'Verily in the remembrance of God do hearts find rest', and 'Therefore remember me, and I will remember you'; and the message, 'Our prayers are with you. In Islam the sick person is closer to God. So remember that the prayer of the sick is good. We will pray for you.'

28th August

A glorious late summer day. A. drives me again up the Woodford Valley. We turn off opposite Sting's mansion in Lake and walk a short way. Huge rolling fields: on one side, wheat awaiting the harvester; on the opposite side, fields of pale-yellow cut straw. Everything glows in a fierce light. Three deer go leaping through the wheat; buzzards call; a scattering of small clouds cast fleeting shadows. Few flowers: the pink and white of bindweed, some purple loosestrife, yellow agrimony, toadflax, autumn hawkbit, blue scabious and a handful of scarlet poppies. Swallows still here. Clumps of dark sycamore, ash and beech break the horizon. All very Wiltshire. Later, watch England win the Fourth Test by a hair's breadth.

Postscript on marriage. John Aubrey, writing of his contemporary George Herbert:

> He married Jane, the third daughter of Charles Danvers ... but had no issue by her. He was a very fine complexion and consumptive. His marriage, I suppose, hastened his death.[44]

Aubrey at his most tantalising.

29th August: Reflecting on wonder (2) and death (1)
Jeremy D. brings us Communion. Judy comes, newly returned from St Petersburg, and recounts the saga of trying to light a candle for me in one of the locked churches. Succeeds at the fourth attempt. Article in today's *Independent* claiming that new scientific research shows that spending time in the countryside is essential to our health. Millions of years in a natural environment have left their mark. We're just not made for high-density urban life. Research shows that residents of a housing estate who live near trees were happier, more sociable and less fearful of crime than those who don't. Patients in hospital who have a view of nature recover quicker than those who stare at brick walls.

In a poem about the desolation of bereavement D. H. Lawrence writes:

> There is nothing to save, now all is lost,
> but a tiny core of stillness in the heart
> like the eye of a violet.[45]

Stillness. Many don't have much opportunity for that, and are starved of (or deny themselves) the healing power of nature. I've written in the past (probably overmuch) about the importance of exercising our capacity for wonder, of opting out for a while from our frenetic hurry-up world into what Keats called the world 'of silence and slow time'. Giving our absorbed attention to what is before our eyes as artists and young children do. Not only because it feeds and nurtures our inner space, but because it is in stillness that we are most open to the numinous, those moments when we begin to sense a hidden Presence in whom we and all that exists 'live and move and have their being'. Which is why prayer needs to be more about stillness, about waiting and listening, than about speaking; recalling who and whose we are. The nature of the extraordinary can strike us in the most seemingly ordinary situations, or when we are contemplating the most apparently ordinary objects. The aim of the artist is to open our eyes to the seeming ordinariness, to its transfiguration.

I wrote the other day that I hoped that as a result of these topsy-turvy weeks when others have been in control of my life, I might discover 'a new simplicity', the ability to stand back from the flow of daily bits and pieces to achieve two things: the recognition of the wonder of the ordinary, and a sense of the whole. To achieve a sense of detachment before the wonder of the world which is lost by our obsession with what the media claim to be important. In his *Memoir* the Irish writer John McGahern attributes his sense of contentment to his upbringing in the remote countryside of the county of Leitrim in north-west Ireland, and his return there 30 years ago. He writes:

> I am sure that it is from those days that I take the belief that the best of life is life lived quietly, where nothing happens but our calm journey through the day, where change is imperceptible and the precious life is everything.[46]

Not that his childhood was idyllic: his mother died of cancer when he was young and his father was an alcoholic who regularly beat his children. (There are echoes there of the poet Edwin Muir, whose idyllic early childhood on an Orkney farm was torn apart when his mother died and his family moved to the slums of Glasgow. At 14 he left school and worked in a factory making fish glue. He spoke of having once had 'one foot in Eden' and all his life searched again for that elusive place.) McGahern writes only of what he knows, what he has experienced and closely observed. Mary Kenny says that 'every word he writes shimmers with integrity'. She describes him as 'a priestly writer in his total commitment and dedication to the religion of the word'.[47] A good analogy. Echoing Auden on suffering, he writes of the world of the dying, of how when accident, stroke or cancer strike, the waitress pouring coffee at table, the builder laying blocks, a girl opening a window, the men collecting refuse, belong to a world that went mainly unregarded when it was ours but now becomes a place of unobtainable happiness, in even the meanest of forms.

'A world that went mainly unregarded.' As we age, we know that death comes a little closer, yet we still put it to the back of our minds. Even when cancer strikes, new treatments no longer mean that its slow poison will spread through the body with a ruthless inevitability. It can be effectively attacked. Nevertheless it reminds you that even if medical advances should enable life to be extended to an unwelcome 200 years, death will come. And you begin to observe the world again with a new passion; with Words-worth's 'listening ear' and Yeats' 'gazing heart'. Not just the people you love and must one day leave, and not just McGahern's ordinary people doing ordinary things which suddenly become enviable, but the sights and sounds and scents of the natural world. It's Walter de la Mare's 'Look thy last on all things lovely'. For me, those lovely things centre on the slowly changing seasons. On the fall of light. The patterns on tree bark. Lichen. The first aconites and snow-drops. A beech tree in May or October. Watching terns diving. Spotting the kingfisher. The view of Mull from the

beach at the north end of Iona; the high pastures coated
with wild flowers in the Tyrol. But it's not just 'looking', but
hearing and tasting and touching too. The sound of swans
flying overhead. The scent of honeysuckle and lilac. The
taste of apricots and the first raspberries. The shapes of
clouds. Swimming in the sea. Listening to music; going to a
theatre or art gallery; reading. The feel of wood and stone;
moulding clay.

In his diary of Devonshire life in the nineteenth and early
twentieth centuries Cecil Torr records an elderly woman in
Lustleigh speaking of her hope of heaven. She told him that
she needed no parsons tò hoist her to heaven, but she was
not in any hurry to get there. 'Looking out across her garden
on a gorgeous summer afternoon, she turned to me, and
said, "I were just a-wonderin' if heaven be so much better
'an this, 'cause, unless it is, I don't know as I'd care for the
change."'[48] I think it was De Quincey who said that death
seemed to him most awful in summer. The American poet,
Peter Kane Dufault, lives and works in a cabin he built
himself deep in the country. He has worked as a tree-
surgeon, journalist, teacher, house-painter, pollster and, in
1968, a candidate for Congress, running on the Liberal
Party's anti-Vietnam war platform. Locally, he's known as a
fiddler, banjo-player, dance-caller – and poet. Here's his
'Evensong':

> Last night when the sun went down
> and the light lifted up – it was levered
> off the last high land westward
> through tier after tier of cirrus
> and cumulus cloud,
> all the way to the zenith – such
> a *finale* of auroral cold fire
> no one could speak here. We stood
> like pillars of salt looking after it
> a long while till it all faded
> into grey and dark-grey. Oh,

how do we survive it, how
do we survive, when more than we dared dream of
is given, for no reason, and for no reason
taken away.[49]

Norman Nicholson once said of the poet/hymn-writer William Cowper of Olney that 'he looks at things with the sharp tenderness of a long goodbye'. 'Sharp tenderness' is good. Sylvia Townsend Warner, best of diarists, writes of the wood-carver and sculptor Reynolds Stone that 'he looks at trees with an astonishing degree of love and trust and penetration; almost as if he were exiled from being a tree himself'.[50] And the spiritual head of the Community of St John on Patmos is quoted in the paper today as saying that 'there is an eleventh commandment: Love the trees. Those who do not love the trees do not love God.'

It's the sense of leaving behind all that is familiar and loved, the small delights as well as the larger joys, that causes us anguish if we are brought face-to-face with the sudden possibility of dying. It makes the deaths of those who have barely tasted life so particularly hard to bear. And we leave all this for what uncertain future? Trust that 'resurrection' is more than just a reassuring word. Carlyle records how a clergyman, 'with surprise, asked Dr Johnson, "Have we not evidence for the soul's immortality?" Samuel Johnson answers, "I wish for more."' Yet if 'resurrection' is no more than a reassuring word, then how do we begin to account for the transformation of the apostles and the rise and embrace of Christianity to contain us? We may wish for more, but in the end it's a question of trust. Trust that the melody endures. My former Cambridge tutor Michael McCrum, who became a close and valued friend, in his small book *Jesus* uses a musical analogy to describe his own personal faith in resurrection:

> Imagine any piece of music that you love. At its creation it was written down by its composer and needed an instrument for its first performance. But once performed it has no further need of

players or instruments. Its particular beauty is in the mind of whoever hears it, just as it was originally in the composer's mind. So, we might be thought to spend our lives as it were composing a piece of music, some more beautiful, some less so, and at our death, when the physical implements which we have used for its composition decay, the music lives on to take its part in the divine orchestration.[51]

Those words were quoted by Mark Pryce last year at Michael's funeral service in the chapel of Corpus Christi, Cambridge, where he had been Master.

So I trust that the God who is the source of my life is not the God of the dead but of the living, that the unique identity that is me will be held in the mind of God and that life in God (which even the most colourful and flowery of images cannot begin to convey) will be rich and fulfilling. John Robinson chose some words of John Donne to be read at his memorial service:

When God loves, he loves to the end; and not to their end, and to their death, but to his end, and his end is that he might love them more.[52]

Even so, however strongly we believe that our relationship with God begins here and now, life in its fulness – life described as 'eternal' because it only rings true if it is somehow analogous to the depth and quality of our best, seemingly timeless, earthly relationships – will always lie on the other side of the dark. And faith would not be faith unless we are prepared to go, naked and trusting, into that darkness and face that final test. Hamlet is right:

There's a special providence in the fall of a sparrow. If it be now, 'tis not to come; if it be not to come, it will be now; if it be not now, yet it will come: the readiness is all.[53]

Another beautiful day. Sit in the garden reading Penelope Lively's *Making It Up*, an autobiographical reflection on the paths not taken, of how life might have been if at certain moments one had taken this path rather than that. As unimaginable as 'heaven', of course, but intriguing. Do I believe that God was guiding me in this direction rather than that at the most important forks in my path? Yes and no. 'No' in the sense that my freedom would have been compromised, suggesting that there was all along only one possible outcome to my life. But 'yes' in the sense that as I tried to pray about these things, whatever guidance came lay in a deepened understanding of myself and my motives, and of where I might best fit and have something useful to share. I also listened to the wise counsel of a few perceptive and trusted friends. Even so: if my father had not taken his life; if my mother had not married again and gone to Africa; if (as I longed to do) I'd gone to RADA and struggled to make a career on the stage; if I'd not met the two men who helped me to come to see that ordination was the only true option; if I'd accepted that tempting job rather than stayed put and subsequently gone to the party where I met A., or resisted those three high-pressure jobs so stubbornly before accepting a fourth; if I hadn't been knocked flat by M.E., or gone to the Abbey ... We all decline so many alternative lives, yet if we're lucky we end up feeling that the life that has been ours had to be the way it was, and we wouldn't wish it otherwise. Only in our dreams do some of the stranger fictions masquerade as reality.

30th August: Reflecting on Jesus (3)

A cloudless day. Judy comes with the catalogue of the Tetryakov Gallery in Moscow, home of the incomparable Rublyev icon of *The Holy Trinity*, made in the 1420s in honour of St Sergius (whose deeply prayerful, unforgettable, candlelit tomb at the monastery of Zagorsk we visited in 1988). Also in the Tetryakov is Rublyev's *The Saviour*, so very damaged, yet still containing the unscathed face of Christ and painted with a touching combination of gravity and grace which was the particular gift of the icon-makers of the fifteenth and sixteenth centuries. It leads me back to Frederick Buechner's richly illustrated book on *The Faces of Jesus* which adds further layers to my search for the 'authentic' Jesus of a few days ago. For his book presents icons of Jesus as the Word made flesh as that universal truth has been interpreted by artists and craftsmen from many different cultures. Each face is different. Some look like Apollo: many are deeply Semitic. These images of the face of Jesus are on gold coins from Byzantium and of his baptism by John in sixth-century mosaics in the Baptistery at Ravenna; in a seventh-century mosaic on the floor of a Dorset church or as the Good Shepherd in the painted first-century Roman catacombs; on Leonardo's *Last Supper* mural in Milan; carved from the polychromed wood of Melanesia and in an Epstein bronze. It is there in the rich silver gilt of fifteenth-century France and on Chinese Christs carved in ivory or embroidered in silk; in works carved in German limestone and walnut and oak; on enamel plaques from Limoges and the carved twelfth-century stone of Autun and Chichester; in illuminated Christs on monastic psalters, solemn Pantocrators from Moscow and St Petersburg, and the angry Temple-cleansing Jesus of El Greco or Rubens' tender *Deposition from the Cross*. There is the scarlet and blue medieval glass of Chartres and Canterbury, and agonised Pietas from Slovenia. Most striking of all is a dark wooden figure of a black Jesus wearing the crown of thorns, carved by an anonymous African craftsman, where the wood speaks, in Buechner's words,

> (of) compassion, beauty, sorrow, majesty, love – as words they are so freighted with meaning that they finally flounder. The wood is mute. What it tells us is simply all there is to tell about what it means to be black, what it means to be a man, what it means to be God.[54]

So we remake the elusive face of Jesus as each new century and different culture recreate him in their own image, even though certain insights remain constant and universal.

Matthias Grunewald's Isenheim altarpiece in Colmar of a cruelly scourged Jesus, his body pock-marked with wounds, no doubt spoke of the kind of plague sores that scarred people's bodies as they were nursed in the adjoining hospice at the time of the Black Death: it speaks just as powerfully to a generation deeply scarred by the Holocaust or (more literally) by the contemporary plague of AIDS. Nor does it matter that we shall never know exactly what Jesus looked like, or that the writers of the New Testament don't describe him. For what mattered to them was no longer his physical presence but the recognition of his life within them. In the words of William Law:

> A Christ not in us is the same thing as a Christ not ours. If ... the history of his title, person and character are all we have of him, we are without him ... It is the language of scripture that Christ in us is our hope of glory, that Christ (being) formed in us, growing and raising his own life and spirit in us, is our only salvation.[55]

The reality is Paul's 'Christ in you, the hope of glory', and his vision of the whole creation being gradually transformed into the 'measure of the stature of the fulness of Christ'. The purpose of life is (in Buechner's words) 'to make Christs of us'. Julian of Norwich wrote: 'Each natural compassion that a man hath on his fellow-Christians with charity, it is Christ in him' (and not simply on 'our fellow-Christians'). We have to combine St John the Divine's majestic image of the Son of Man in the heavenly Jerusalem whose face is 'like the sun shining in full strength', and – more modestly – Jesus' claim that wherever we serve the hungry, the poor, the needy and the sick, we are serving him. The reality is the Sisters of the Missionaries of Charity in Calcutta gently washing each of the bodies of the dying newly carried in from the streets under a simple sign proclaiming 'The body of Christ'. It is Turgenev dreaming of kneeling in a wooden Orthodox church where slim wax candles gutter in front of icons. A

man comes and stands behind him and all at once he senses
that this man is Christ.

> It was a face like everyone's, a face like all men's faces ... the
> hands folded and still, the clothes like everyone's. 'What sort of
> Christ is this?' I thought. 'Such an ordinary, ordinary man! It
> can't be!' (He turns away, but his eyes are drawn back to the
> figure beside him.) And suddenly my heart sank, and I came to
> myself. Only then did I realise that just such a face – a face like
> all men's faces – is the face of Christ.[56]

In bed listen to a Haydn Mass and read Robert Harris' *Pompeii*. An odd mix.

31st August

Card from Tim and Pru West showing the 1911 ballot of the
Actresses' Franchise League, formed 'to convince members
of the theatrical profession of the necessity of extending the
franchise to women'. Today is in fact the twenty-fifth
anniversary of the rise of Solidarity in Poland, also the result
of union action which led the people finally to throw off the
Communist yoke. Recall Lech Welesa, trade union leader
turned President, coming to the Abbey with his wife and
(uniquely among visiting heads of state) falling to their
knees before the altar in Edward the Confessor's shrine, and
saying their prayers.

Drive again to Lake and walk a few yards further. See
heron, and hares dozing in the cut fields. Too hot to write.

1st September

Wake each morning to a view of the backs of terraced houses
200 yards away, and beyond them, on the skyline, the
magnificent copper beeches and horse chestnut in Bourne
Gardens, with, rising above them, the slim spire of the
cathedral with its metal cross: a pleasing mix of the human,
the natural and the transcendent.

Reflecting on suffering

A thousand lie dead and hundreds are injured in a panicking crowd of pilgrims in Baghdad; hundreds are dead and New Orleans devastated by Hurricane Katrina; and S. comes and tells me of her nephew, diagnosed in his mid thirties with stomach cancer. How can I think it matters to write about my own time of testing, so trivial when compared with that of so many? How would my faith stand up to such a sense of gut-wrenching desolation? None of us knows until we are in a similar situation what resources of courage and faith we may possess. And yet: Christianity has its roots in the anguish of Gethsemane, and in the blood and pain of Calvary. Easter doesn't erase that most passionate of human cries: 'My God, *why* have you forsaken me?' even if St John's Gospel asserts that it is followed by the triumphant claim, 'It is accomplished!' and (according to Luke) by the absolute trust of 'Into your hands I commend my spirit.' The Christian faith was born from the conviction of those who knew him best that Jesus – mysteriously but unquestionably – was alive in their midst, reassuring and empowering them to face with courage and with trust whatever might come. And what came, and has continued to come whenever the Gospel has been lived out with that passion for truth and justice that questions and provokes those who exercise earthly power, has continued to be costly: at times, persecution and imprisonment, even martyrdom. That's why the west front of Westminster Abbey now contains ten figures of twentieth-century martyrs, standing between figures symbolising truth, justice, mercy and peace.

'Does my Creator weep?' Jesus weeps at the grave of Lazarus. He heals the sick, reassuring them that neither sickness nor accidents like the crushing of people in a collapsing building (the tower of Siloam) are sent by God, but that God may be found within the experience; in God's name he forgives the sinful, and goes to his death in order to show the ultimate powerlessness of the kind of worldly authority (be it the aggression of Rome or the inhumane face of

Communism or military juntas) which would use power to twist and control the human spirit and gainsay its freedom. At first his ministry, as a rabbi, is to the Jews: it ends, in its implications, by being addressed to all humanity – as Paul quickly understood when Peter did not. Our inborn instinct to be self-seeking causes all of us to fall short of what we are created to be: those created in Love's likeness and acting in Love's language. But Christians are not alone in believing in a compassionate God, and that's why whenever acts of prayer and remembrance are held – after 9/11, the bomb outrages in London, or other acts of terror – Muslim, Jewish and Christian leaders come together and speak with a united voice.

Every human being has the right to compassionate action and concern. That's why Amnesty candles now burn in many cathedrals and churches, and why prisoners of conscience (of all faiths and none) are prayed for daily at thousands of Eucharists. That's why Salisbury Cathedral is dominated by the radiant east window showing the light from the central figure on the Cross illuminating the faces of such prisoners. Once you believe that Jesus, in his attentive doing of the Father's will that inevitably leads to the dereliction of Calvary, is our truest, most valid window into God, a heartrending image of that power which (in Paul's words) is shown most perfectly in weakness, then you hear that twisted body on the Cross declaring once and for all time: 'Yes, our Creator weeps.' Weeps as we weep. Not just at the human readiness to oppress and cause each other pain, but also at the inevitable weakness which mortality implies, as we succumb to pain and suffering when body or mind malfunctions, or death intervenes.

The daily evidence and heartbreaking consequences of this dual freedom – to cause hurt or to be hurt – lead many to reject God. Others find their faith tested to the limit, for faith worthy of the name will be a tried and questioning faith if it is to hold firm in the dark. In response to Milton's declared aim in *Paradise Lost* to 'assert eternal Providence/ And justify the ways of God to man', Housman wrote the ironic couplet: '... malt does more than Milton can,/ to justify the ways of God to man'. That's an understandable response to the death of tens of thousands of young men in war, but like all jibes it doesn't satisfy. In seeking answers to the enigma of suffering we have to accept that we have limited powers. Eliot's 'hints and guesses'. Yet tested over time by countless people (four of whom are the dedicatees of this book); those who have found strength and courage in extremity by believing that 'I may go down to hell, but thou art there also.' 'Thou': not William Blake's 'Nobodaddy', remote and removed from his creation, but the Christlike God. If this is simply wishful thinking, if we are merely the product of random evolutionary processes, it is just as hard intellectually to account for those uniquely human qualities of courage and grace, altruism, empathy, and a yearning for the good to prevail, that seem to be deeply ingrained in all but the most damaged of human hearts – irrespective of whether or not those who display such qualities accept the reality of God in their lives. Like the wind, the Spirit blows where it wills and signs of the 'Kingdom-heart' are found in unexpected people and places. For that's the privilege we enjoy in being free spirits. And any other option would not be the invitation to encounter and respond to a God of love. It would be the response of a carefully programmed computer, ringed around and safeguarded from disasters or mistakes. As incapable of loving as of causing hurt.

However, to return to my starting-point, even though when compared with sickness or suffering at its most testing my own troubles may be very small beer, in the end I can only tell bits of my own story and hope that bits of it will resonate with bits of yours. I may not be able to understand exactly what you are experiencing, but the least I can do is to listen. For surely the things that can be shared more than compensate for all the things that can't.

Walk by the Avon. A strong feel of late summer. Robins singing, coots fussing about, little grebe diving. Willow-herb, gypsywort, common fleabane, growing by the banks. In the evening watch John Huston's adaptation of one of the finest short stories in the language: James Joyce's *The Dead*.

2nd September

To the clinic this morning. I.D., back from holiday, seems pleased with my agonisingly slow progress. We are to meet next week to discuss radiotherapy. A cloudless day.

Reflecting on 'being Church' (1)

Writing yesterday of the test of faith in the face of dereliction, I spoke of human grace and courage, deliberately not distinguishing between 'human' and 'Christian', and of the 'Kingdom-heart', though without speaking of the place of the Church. The latter, of course, only makes sense when understood as the agent of the far broader concept of the Kingdom. The great Russian theologian Nicholas Berdyaev once wrote:

> There are two symbols, bread and money; and there are two mysteries, the eucharistic mystery of bread and the Satanic mystery of money. We are faced with the great task: to over-throw the rule of money and to establish in its place the rule of bread.[57]

Just as Baptism (together with the Eucharist) creates and defines the Church, so the Church's task is to define the true meaning of community. We need to distinguish between religion and spirituality. Religion, where authentic, embraces the spiritual, but 'spirituality' is much wider than religion. It has come to stand for that which relates to the human spirit, and seeks meaning and significance in the whole of human experience. We may reject Bono's remark that 'religion is what is left when the Spirit has left the building', even if in many cases that seems undeniable: churches where the liturgy has become tired, clergy who feel dispirited and defeated, some like Samson with his locks shorn as he slept and his strength gone, 'and he knew it not'. Yet the fashion for a kind of DIY, 'I-did-it-my-way' spirituality, so evident in all the 'mind, body, spirit' sections of the larger bookshops, or a Glastonbury almost entirely given over to shops whose names play variations on 'The Psychic Piglet', is in direct opposition to any traditional expresssion of the Gospel or of worship. Individualism has no place in Christianity. It's true that central to any Christian understanding is an emphasis on the unique and infinite worth of every human being, but only if that is held in balance with the claim that we escape our aloneness in the adventure of love and friendship. We need each other in order that we may become ourselves. It sees us exploring our potential as lovers-in-the-making within the context of the new creation where, in Martin Buber's words, 'everything is a Thou and nothing is an It'.

From the start Christianity has portrayed itself as offering the world a new model of human community. So the New Testament is not so much concerned with the private interior life of the individual, but with our new shared humanity in Christ and the building up of the local body of believers as one cell in the infinitely greater body of all who have sought, and all who now seek, to centre their lives on him. Its marks are faith expressed as worship and love expressed in action, what Rowan Williams has called 'a community of those so overwhelmed by their indebtedness to God's free grace that they live in a state of glad and grateful indebtedness to one another'.

At least in theory. The figures for the percentage of the population attending a weekly religious service are: Denmark 2%, Germany 11%, UK, Spain, Belgium and the Netherlands 16%, Italy 31%, Poland 54%. But that tells us nothing about whether those who dismiss the Church do so because they don't believe in God, or because of a bad experience, or because of a wildly mistaken concept of Christian belief, or for a variety of other reasons. No one denies the constant failure of the Church throughout history to be a true representative of Christ's body on earth. Time and again it has 'called the green leaf grey', lost its vision, denied or betrayed Jesus as Peter and Judas did, refused to go the second mile, become deeply worldly, joined with relish in the crucifying of the good, the innocent and those who stand for truth. It has stifled the Spirit, turning the passion and radicalism of the Gospel into a bland and complacent gathering of the like-minded where Morning Prayer wends its beautiful but undemanding way, or where bread and wine happen to be on the menu this Sunday rather than coffee and biscuits. One can take the admirable Anglican qualities of moderation and a seeking of 'the middle way' to absurd extremes. It has been written off

> by many of those in every nation who care most for social justice and the fashioning of a humaner life ... We need to acknowledge a pride, a lust for power, a cynicism, an insensitiveness to human suffering which went far to alienate the oppressed people of the earth ... and which made much of its spirituality stink in the nostrils of the Lord God of all the earth.[58]

None of this is surprising. The Church of God is made up of damaged, fallible human beings. Yet such aberrations of what the Church is called to be, though useful weapons with which its opponents can rubbish her, do nothing to invalidate the vision, any more than a messy divorce invalidates marriage. They don't negate the reality of the Christian way as that has been lived out by the Desert Fathers, the members of monastic communities, by those ordinary, extraordinary individuals we call 'saints', and by assemblies of people in every age and from every nation and tradition as they seek together to open their lives to Christ. And in so doing, by pondering on the word and gathering in every conceivable circumstance and need in order to share the eucharistic bread, they have entered (as we now enter) into the story of God acting in history to initiate his Kingdom. When we worship we take our place with those first-century

146

Christians who met in one another's houses to celebrate the Resurrection of Jesus in the breaking of bread and, like them, go out to live lives which are subtly altered by what we have done together.

Today the talk is of how Church may most effectively 'be Church' to a generation suspicious of the word, yet intrigued by the transcendent and hungry for the 'something more' of the spiritual. It's hard for those of us trained in a tradition that (unwisely perhaps) took so much God-language for granted to find new ways of clothing truths which have become part of us. Yet (as I wrote in Part I) I know that any enduring melody must contain all that is signified by that shared meal. It has been the way Christians have linked time and eternity as, day by day, Sunday by Sunday, they have recalled the death of Jesus, the ultimate sacrifice that a man can make for others, whose meaning has nothing to do with God's 'wrath' but everything to do with his love; and with the drama that was completed three days later in the garden and the upper room. It makes present again that Last Supper where Jesus, taking the bread, giving thanks for it, breaking and sharing it, identifies it with his life, identifies it with the whole self-giving, dying-to-self pattern of it which was now to be their pattern (and hence *our* pattern) too. Here is the body language of God come into our midst. It looks forward to the time when the Kingdom-heart will have triumphed and the 'eucharistic mystery of bread' becomes the norm in our scandalously unequal world, where now every cow in the European Union is subsidised to the tune of $2.50 a day, and a billion people round the world struggle to live on $1 a day. It is a *political* statement, deeply incarnational. It is the most earthy and materialistic of sacraments. And by moving forward and holding out our hands to receive the broken bread, having yet again received forgiveness for our failure to live lives reliant on God's grace, we are desiring, choosing, to be identified with the costly way of love. And that is *being* Church. And it's no easier when you're 80 than it was when you were 18.

The shape of the ordained ministry has changed and will no doubt continue to do so. There will be women bishops. Patterns of worship will grow more flexible. The Anglican Communion may break apart over questions of gender. But I pray that Anglicanism may remain sufficiently true to itself to bring one day to a truly united Church the gifts of tolerance and inclusiveness, and the recognition that truth may lie in seemingly irreconcilable extremes. These have been among its most precious marks; and that fourfold pattern of the Eucharist which has shaped the liturgical life of the great traditions of Orthodoxy, Roman Catholicism, Anglicanism, and those that sprang up out of the seeds of the Reformation, will still be the recognisable sign of those who call themselves Christians in the unimaginable centuries ahead.

Reading Sydney Smith, residentiary canon of St Paul's Cathedral. In addition, in 1828, he was made prebend of Bristol Cathedral. He was astonished at how small his clerical colleagues were:

> It is supposed that one of the ecclesiastics elevated upon the shoulders of the other, should fall short of the summit of the Archbishop of Canterbury's wig ... The Archbishop of York is forced to go down on his knees to converse with the Bishop of Bristol, just as an elephant receives its rider.

The meetings of the Chapter of St Paul's must have been greatly enlivened by his presence.

3rd–4th September: Reflecting on 'being Church' (2)
Yesterday's thoughts should have ended with a colon, for there's more to be said. Though perhaps not by the elderly. We tend to be bewildered when what we have spent our lives defending seems to be crumbling, partly today through a generational distrust of institutions, be they monarchy, Parliament, or Church. The young have always tended to break free from a prescribed set of dogmatic imperatives or

to challenge afresh inherited structures. Each new generation has the right to interrogate the tradition it inherits if it
is to remain healthy. Jesus, both creative and subversive,
certainly questioned his own, observing the Mosaic code,
but challenging it. The Jewish faith and Scriptures were his
life-blood, and that enabled him to speak from within the
tradition, to criticise its stifling legalism and point people to
those unheeded truths about the nature of God and the
implications of his sovereignty which the prophets had
known, but which had been overlaid by conservative forces
who had lost the plot and made religion not merely complicated but boring. 'Is it a small thing for you to weary men,
but will you weary my God also?'[59] His words carried an
authority, a persuasiveness, that not only liberated those
who heard them but have somehow survived the turmoil of
the centuries and still have the power to do so.

Rowan Williams is among those who are committed to
new ways of 'being Church', the in-phrase of the moment.
But a good one, with its reminder that the word 'church'
loses its power when applied to buildings rather than to
people: people who have been called, in Paul's potent
phrase, 'to put on the Lord Jesus Christ', we in him, he in us.
Slowly shaped, changed, renewed, in the long journey of
love and its meaning. Yet this isn't how it strikes those who
dip their toes into the water. Too often they find con-
gregations which are small and grey-haired, the worship
somewhere on a graph between 'bland' and 'complacent'.
Too often they look in vain for that element of stillness and
silence which allows for the possibility of something more,
an openness to the 'Beyond in our midst', the numinous
Mystery. Or there seems little sense of addressing at any
depth human need or conveying a sense of the challenging
values of the Kingdom. Too often the intercessions take the
form of reminding God of the news of the day and adding a
quick shopping-list of what we think we need but sense we
are unlikely to get. (Which, of course, is true, unless we are
prepared to think through our real priorities and engage

them with the necessary desire.) That may not be as true of the growing body of evangelical churches where there is lively worship (where it hasn't tipped over into a form of emotional self-indulgence) and large numbers of people under 40 – though not always much space or stillness. Nor of the Pentecostal tradition, the fastest-growing in the world. Nor, in terms of imaginative worship reaching across the divide of the traditions and the generations, of a centre like Taizé. But the spirit of Taizé is not easily transposed; and many of us are by temperament and upbringing somewhat shy and uneasy with the freer, less restrained and structured worship of evangelicals and charismatics, and chary of a theology that (in its more conservative form) tends to be too neatly boxed and unquestioned.

There are other traditions, faithful to aspects of Jesus' teaching, other forms of spirituality, such as that of the gentle Quakers (or, better, the Society of Friends, empha-sising the corporate and shared) who reject any formal ministry, ritual or sacraments, but who have refused to take part in war and in any kind of personal violence, though they have been among the first to organise relief for its victims and showed courage in sending ambulance units into the battlefield. They took the lead in abolishing slavery and worked for prison reform and better education. All actions close to the heart of Jesus. I admire them greatly, yet I can't deny my heritage. I have loved the Church of Eng-land and its sometimes bizarre ways. I can't imagine feeling at home in any other tradition (nor in the extreme fringes of Anglicanism). As layman and priest there have been experiences of worship, often at the great festivals or in Holy Week but equally at early celebrations of the Eucharist with a tiny handful of people present, which have been among the most valued experiences of my life. Not so much because they have brought some mystical experience of God, but because they have carried the conviction that what we are celebrating are the tested truths of what it means to respond to a God who is vulnerable and near at hand and of yourself and everyone else as potentially Christlike. When that happens through an act of worship, it really feels celebratory: a small light illuminating the darkness and redressing the balance. For 60 years I have shared in the breaking of bread, not always very devotionally, but more often than not with a sense of coming home, of the rightness of belonging to these people in this place. A priest is privileged to share in so many people's joys and sorrows and – with a very few challenging exceptions – when you do that you grow to love them.

I was trained in a tradition in which word and sacrament are finely balanced, where worship is well and thoughtfully ordered, where (hopefully) head matches heart in a single integrity. And for nearly half my life I worshipped using the incomparable words of the King James' Bible and the rich, if historically dated, prose of the *Book of Common Prayer*, born from the new needs of the post-Reformation Church. Having lived through the changes, I can understand the yearning of members of the Prayer Book Society for the old and the familiar, even while I welcome the new insights of scholars and liturgies – some of which are very fine – that more realistically meet the needs of our time. But there remains the question of how we meet equally the needs of the older generation with real understanding while new ways of 'being Church' are explored. That needs patience and sensitivity and there are no easy answers. Yet transition is inevitable. It's how the world ticks. And if we're wise, we take what endures because other ages have valued and preserved it and seek to hold fast to it even where that means reclothing it in words and actions which attempt to speak to our own age of the transcendent nature of truth, the beauty of holiness, and the winning love of God.

Another phrase being banded about among those who worry over the Church's future in a profoundly changed society is 'believing, not belonging'. Though just how much, and just what, the 70 per cent of the population who still tick the census form in the space marked 'Christian' but rarely enter a place of worship, actually believe is anyone's guess. Like all generalisations, it's a very rough guide. But research shows that many, especially the young, don't have problems with believing in God (however conceived) but with belonging. They are chronic 'non-joiners'. It's not simply that our traditional style of expressing what we believe isn't their style, but that institutions which are slow to adapt to change are viewed with impatience. Nor do they share our vocabulary. Yet listen to the young and you may find a quality of awareness of other people, a passionate concern for international justice, an impatience with the slow response to issues of poverty, and a growing sense of stewardship for the earth and responsibility for each other that put to shame the narrow, more domestic interests that many of us shared 50 years ago, as well as a lot of the current domestic concerns of the Church. And many put their money where their mouth is. Social work in the community is part of the timetable of many schools. Volunteering to work in the Third World in their gap year is increasingly common. Many who feel a hunger to explore the life of the spirit yet find mainstream churches inadequate or unshifting bastions of certainty look elsewhere. Some turn to more rarefied New Age rites that appear to allow for greater freedom. Others revert to the earliest pattern of meeting in house churches for a more intimate form of fellowship.

Yet if by 'being Church' we mean holding true to the tradition, that shouldn't imply blind conformity, weighed down by the heavy baggage of the past. Throughout history monopolistic claims to divine truth have eventually transmuted into the poison of anti-Semitism, conflict in Northern Ireland, the Islamic suicide bombers and executioners, and even the justification of genocide. Neither Muslim, Christian nor Jew can claim a monopoly of truth when it comes to approaching the Supreme Being. Even the Christian claim that God was in Christ enabling us to catch an authentic glimpse of the Love that lies at the heart of things is held in tension with the truth that 'my thoughts are not your thoughts', that ultimately God can't be comprehended, only apprehended. Any attempt to domesticate him, to create a God in *our* image rather than coming to see that we are made in his, is bound to fail. This isn't to say that God becomes a kind of *terra incognita*. When Bonhoeffer talks of God as 'the Beyond' he qualifies that by speaking of 'the Beyond *in our midst*'. As well as being the *alpha* and *omega* of the human drama, its beginning and its end, he is found at the very heart of it. Further, no human institution, no book written by men (however 'inspired'), has copyright of the truth, neither the Jewish Scriptures, the New Testament, the Koran, the Upanishads and the Bhagavadgita of Hinduism, or the Guru Granth of Buddhism. In the face of the Mystery whom we call God we should be careful not to claim too much. 'Both read the Bible day and night,' writes William Blake, 'But thou reads't black where I read white.'[60] Whatever faith we follow in our search for the numinous and the transcendent, it is one that can never claim to grasp the truth entire, but which recognises the need to add the words of Oliver Cromwell to the General Assembly of the Church of Scotland: 'I beseech you, in the bowels of Christ, think it possible that you may be mistaken.'

This is not to water down 'the enduring melody', the gold that remains when the dross has been sifted away and which may be tested by fire when called upon to resist evil, or when cancer strikes and the icy threat of dying seems closer than it did before. It is simply to be honest about our limitations when the best we can hope for is to see through a glass darkly, to live with a certain ambiguity, to 'tell the truth, but tell it slant'. To have faith is to explore – and go on exploring – the life of the spirit on the only journey that matters: that of becoming a more rounded and authentic human being. It is to expose yourself to what has been thought of most value by past generations and test it in the light of your experience in the present. In the words of Father Gerard Hughes: 'If the critical element is not fostered, Christians will remain infantile in their religious belief and

153

practice, which will bear little relation to everyday life and behaviour.' To be continued ...

5th September: Reflecting on 'being Church' (3)

So what must 'being Church' mean if it is to meet the needs of the age in which our grandchildren are growing up? It will mean creating spaces in which people may catch a glimpse of the awesome holiness of God as well as the mystery of his vulnerability and compassion. It will seek to express the traditional quintessence of the Gospel in ways that satisfy the intellect as well as the heart: using words and employing images and metaphors which speak to both but which also speak where reason runs out of words. Like art and poetry and drama and falling in love, it will demand a combination of intelligence and feeling. It will mean stilling the demand that we should sign up to some credal formulary, allowing people who have always found themselves in that borderland between faith and scepticism to go on exploring, but *within*, not outside, the worshipping community. It will mean loving God's world, but learning to stand obliquely to the traffic of values dictated by the media and the consumerist world of self-interest, learning to redress the balance with the Gospel values of forgiveness, reconciliation, empathy, equity and self-denying love. The eucharistic mystery of bread as opposed to the satanic mystery of money.

'Being Church' means celebrating and building on people's natural kindness and goodness, affirming human beings in their aloneness and pointing to the God who not only understands and shares their times of darkness but also lies on the other side of the dark. But it will not be 'Church' at all unless it is made up of a gathered community where *believing implies belonging*, finding its fragile unity in the only reason for its existence: to be slowly shaped in the likeness of our Creator, the pattern of Jesus Christ. It will always be full of frail human beings struggling to live in harmony. The miracle is that there is a hidden melody traceable in the teaching of Jesus and the insights of Paul which has survived all the radical challenges of history. Survived not just those corrruptions of the Gospel that have so frequently seen Christians favour law over grace, worldly power over the way of the servant-king, the persecution of other faiths rather than a recognition of their insights, and an unattractive exclusivity and judgementalism over inclusivity and dialogue. It has shown an impressive ability to change its spots while (just) retaining its integrity as each new age responds to social and cultural shifts, and to the ever-steeper learning curve in its grasp of the creation, its laws and its creatures.

For consider: by the second century Christians formed a kind of secret society, their baptism disallowing them to offer sacrifices to the Emperor. They met on the first day of the week to sing hymns, to commit themselves to the two pivotal laws of loving God and loving neighbour, and to share in a simple meal centred on the breaking of bread. For two-and-a-half centuries they struggled to survive. Many were martyred. Only when the Emperor Constantine embraced the Christian faith did the persecution stop and was the Church set free to define its central beliefs. The Roman Empire, which stretched from Scotland to Libya, Portugal to Iraq, became the Holy Roman Empire. (Although the people weren't exactly given the choice of believing. In 998 in Kiev, when Prince Vladimir adopted Christianity, he ordered the citizens to undergo a mass baptism in the River Dnieper.) With the decline of the Empire and the invasion of the barbarians the only institution to preserve elements of law and order was the Church, largely through the monasteries which originated in Egypt in the fourth century for those seeking a celibate and ascetic life. In Britain, by the end of the third century, the Celtic church was beginning to be established. It was practically extinguished 200 years later by the coming of the Saxons but small pockets survived in remote parts. Then in the sixth century Columba of Iona and Aidan of Lindisfarne, with their small monastic and missionary communities, began to transform it, and it rapidly grew. With the coming of Augustine to establish a form of the Roman church the Irish-inspired Celtic church of the north found itself at odds with Christians in the south until at the Synod of Whitby the choice fell on Rome.

During the Dark Ages in Europe, the centuries leading up to the millennium, it was only the humane influence of the monasteries which kept the faith alive. They laid the foundation for learning and education, and they continued to exercise formidable power. In Britain the reform movement in the late tenth century under Ethelwold, Dunstan and Oswald, enabled the monasteries to reach uniformity under the common Rule of St Benedict. The Middle Ages saw a kind of golden age for the Church: powerful monasteries, the building of the great Gothic cathedrals, the establishment of the systems of law and administration, impressive scholarship. Europe and Christendom were synonymous entities. The result? A Church deeply compromised by its collusion with worldly powers. The Papacy was dangerously powerful, the Roman church steeped in abuse and corruption. (Henry VIII's Chancellor, Cardinal Wolsey, had a mistress by whom he had a son whom he made, while still a schoolboy, Dean of Wells.) So much worldly power inevitably contained seeds of its own decay. In Britain Henry VIII laid waste the hugely powerful monasteries, seizing their land and goods for himself. But all over Europe the demand for reform was erupting. A new theological dynamic saw Zwingli, Calvin and, above all, Martin Luther, preaching a Gospel which taught that salvation came, not through the doing of good works, but simply by responding to the sheer grace of the love and forgiveness of God revealed in Jesus. In Cambridge, centre of reform, Erasmus, Matthew Parker, Ridley, Latimer and Cranmer (the latter three to be martyred under the Catholic Queen Mary) led a scholarly revival of the English church. Henry, having suppressed the monasteries, ordered the Bible in English to be set up in all churches. Where once the study of the Bible had been the

156

preserve of religious houses and scholars, now, with the invention of printing, folk could possess their own copy and read it at home in the vernacular. Owen Chadwick writes of how 'the brazier, the felt-maker and the coachman – the working people – went into the Bible to fetch their divinity for themselves'.[61] But it was only with the accession of Elizabeth, with her aversion to extremes and the urgent need to reach some reconciliation between Papists and Puritans (those who still looked to Rome and emphasised ritual and the sacramental life, and those who looked to Luther's 'by faith alone' and Calvin's desire for plainness), that a comprehensive settlement was reached. It can't have been easy for tender consciences to adapt to married clergy and services in English. I'm reading Ronan Bennett's fine novel *Havoc, In the Third Year*,[62] about Catholic recusants in Yorkshire and the Puritan-led fanatics who hunted them down and half-hanged, then disembowelled, the priests. A reminder of the terrible cost to hundreds of good men and women of the eventual triumph of a national church created by Cranmer, Laud, John Jewel and Richard Hooker, who saw the church as an *organic, developing body within an organic, changing society*; some of the speakers in General Synod would do well to remember this. Those who protested against the corruption of the Church of Rome and those whose secret Catholic faith continued to sustain them (often at great cost) gradually learned to live together in a reformed church which was at once a continuation of the old and familiar and a new, inevitably slow, messy and violent transmutation as the defining marks of the Church of England became established. Here was a distinctive way of 'being Church' that was to become an Anglican Communion consisting of 75 million members in 165 countries.

I'm no historian, but even this absurdly potted version of Church history reveals that today's upheavals over the role of women and gender, and the challenge to find new ways of 'being Church' which are consonant with the Gospel are as nothing compared with the upheavals of the past. There is a certain arrogance if we claim to live in uniquely troubled times, and a lack of faith in doubting that the authentic Christian melody (not least in its Anglican guise) will endure. 'History', said Bishop Lightfoot of Durham in 1873, 'is an excellent cordial for drooping spirits.' The Church of England survived the languors of the eighteenth century when it nearly died of boredom, the challenges of biblical scholarship in the nineteenth century, together with Charles Darwin's theory of evolution (which I have sought to show in *Learning to Dance* in no way compromises an intelligent view of God as Creator); and even Matthew Arnold's 'melancholy, long withdrawing roar' of the sea of faith.

Jesus promised his disciples that 'the Spirit of truth would lead (them) into all truth'. Whatever the future holds, I am constantly glad to belong to a church which at its best seeks to be open to that Spirit, able to contain within it people of profoundly different views, finding its strength not in some bland uniformity but in something much more precious and true to the Gospel: unity in diversity. At its worst, it has seen God as a rather superior, decent, beneficent English squire of a well-ordered universe reflected in a well-ordered society, 'the rich man in his castle, the poor man at his gate'. Somerset Maugham recalled going to stay with the diarist Augustus Hare at Herstmonceaux in 1898. There was formal Morning Prayer each day for the servants, and Maugham noticed that the prayers used by Hare from the *Book of Common Prayer* had been severely edited. When questioned Hare replied:

> I've crossed out all the passages in glorification of God. God is certainly a gentleman, and no gentleman cares to be praised to his face. It is tactless, impertinent and vulgar. I think all that fulsome adulation must be highly offensive to him.[63]

At its best, the Church of England seeks to hold together in a creative and dynamic tension a *catholic* understanding of the continuity of the Church and the central place within it of the sacraments of Baptism and Eucharist; an *evangelical* understanding of the importance of the word of God, of personal conversion and the centrality of the cross; and a truly *liberal* freedom of thought and conscience, with a desire to serve individuals, whoever they may be and whatever their need. Whether or not they believe and whether or not they belong.

At times of national mourning (the death of Princess Diana, a ferry disaster, a bomb outrage, the murder of children), and however mixed their motives, people still need to express their grief and concern within a church or cathedral setting. Only ten days ago Liverpool Cathedral was packed to the doors for the funeral of a murdered black teenager, all his contemporaries dressed (at his mother's request) in football shirts. Just as our churches will be packed each Christmas for carol services and midnight mass. And then there are memorial services. Three years ago, the journalist Will Hutton, writing in the *Observer* of a memorial service for a former news editor at St Bride's, Fleet Street, for those who 'wanted to spend an hour to honour a man we respected and loved' (and) 'notably in church', described how

> few in a secular age manage a deep-felt commitment to religious faith, but once again the Church of England had opened its doors to a group of scarcely religious people with whom it had the slightest of relationships but who needed the combination of shrine and liturgy to express a deep appreciation of someone they had loved and lost ... (This) openness is but one component of a relaxed, profoundly tolerant faith that accepts our fallibilities and which is fundamentally reassuring at moments of loss. Our collective relationship with the Church of England runs very deep. I concede my attachment to the church is as much cultural, attracted by its inclusiveness, kindness and tolerance, as any faith I may have. It represents, for all its weakness, the best of England. It is about being open to everyone in all their imperfect and sometimes non-existent relationship with faith.[64]

Relaxed; open; inclusive; kind; tolerant. I'll settle for that.

6th September

To Southampton Hospital to see the oncology consultant Chris Baughan, who will monitor my six weeks of radiotherapy. A senior consultant, who taught my surgeon I.D., drops by to inspect the latter's work in my mouth and declares himself both impressed and a touch jealous. He warns me that I may feel low in the coming weeks, not to put on a brave face but to let my emotions emerge, not to be afraid of tears. Unlikely that a senior consultant of even ten years ago would have expressed such views. An encouraging shift. An analogy there, perhaps, to our coming to terms with change in the Church. Here is a man trained in a different medical tradition, prepared to adapt to new insights about how his profession most effectively communicates with patients and seeks, not just to convey a sense of confidence in its medical skills, but to address them as persons at every level, body, mind and spirit.

C.B. is joined by I.D. They explain what is to happen. In two weeks I shall be fitted with a plastic mask and radiotherapy will start three weeks later. As I.D. had warned me, the cancer in one of the removed lymph glands had spread into another, just beneath the left ear. As I understand it, if left alone, it would then gradually creep down the neck, as down the rungs of a ladder. The radiation will be aimed at an area covering the left side of the neck, part of the tongue and throat and jaw. It will cause burning and tenderness and it will be cumulative. The few remaining saliva glands will cease to work properly and the saliva become sluggish and unpleasant. I may lose my taste. There is no certainty that the cancer will not return but this is the most effective way to prevent it from doing so. There will be exhaustion and a possibility of the return of M.E. The six-and-a-half weeks of daily sessons 'will prove as demanding as the operation'. So be it.

160

Very weary as the result of the 45-minute drive to Southampton and the hour-and-three-quarters spent there.

7th September

To town for the first time where I sign on for a Shopmobility electric three-wheeled scooter, £1 a day, maximum speed 4 m.p.h. Given a driving lesson in the car park, then visit the Playhouse where I'm chaplain (heart-warming welcome) and Ottakar's bookshop to stock up for the coming months. In the garden roses vie with unseasonal primroses.

8th September

This morning I watch our sole and shapely old apple tree being cut down, feeling like Firs at the end of Chekhov's *The Cherry Orchard*, though modern chainsaws are rather more brutal than that slow, haunting thwack of the axe as the curtain falls in the play. The stump will remain, too large to remove. Over these nine years, while I've sat by the window, it has given such pleasure, as well as an annual crop of somewhat wormy apples. No longer now a lodging place for tits, goldfinch and siskin, and the resident pair of collared doves.

Thinking further about the implications of Christians bonded together by sharing in the Eucharist, Alice Meynell's poem, 'The Unknown God', comes to mind. It begins:

> One of the crowd went up,
> And knelt before the Paten and the Cup,
> Received the Lord, returned in peace, and prayed
> Close to my side. Then in my heart I said:
>
> O Christ, in this man's life –
> This stranger who is Thine – in all his strife,
> All his felicity, his good and ill,
> In the assaulted stronghold of his will,
>
> I do confess Thee here
> Alive within this life ...

Christ in his numbered breath,
Christ in his beating heart and in his death,
Christ in his mystery! ...[65]

That great parish priest, Alan Ecclestone, father of my one-time colleague Giles (one of the dedicatees of this book), reflecting on that poem and on his experience of 'going to a new church where everyone was still unknown to me', writes:

It is easy to half-acknowledge and not to notice that the Christ is in them. It is humbling too for the one who has presided at the Holy Communion to look out at the people on leaving the altar, to look on Christ embodied. In which direction should one bow?[66]

Manage to gather blackberries at Charlton All Saints, but still feel pretty drained. Watch Bruckner's Eighth Symphony from the Proms. New moon and Venus crystal-clear half-an-hour after sunset.

9th September

Three members of one of the still active prayer-groups I launched 25 years ago at Great St Mary's send me the handsome catalogue of the current exhibition at Cambridge's Fitzwilliam Museum of ten centuries of illuminated books. It chimes with my words of a couple of days ago about the monasteries' role in keeping burning the flame of faith from the end of the Dark Ages to the Reformation. The earliest is the illuminated Gospels from the sixth century brought by St Augustine when he was sent to England by the Pope. Beautifully embellished Gospel Books and Psalters are most common before the twelfth century, with an increasing enthusiasm for scenes from the Apocalypse and Lives of the Saints in the thirteenth and fourteenth, and by the fifteenth century the more personal Books of Hours, containing the daily Offices of the Breviary. Many of the devotional books have borders decorated with wild flowers, butterflies, snails, lions and monkeys, peacocks, goldfinch, beetles, worms. Not all of them are for liturgical or devotional purposes: some illustrate the known sciences of arithmetic, music, geometry and astronomy. A few include personifications of the planets, a zodiac, maps of the imagined, unexplored world. Some are Bestiaries showing real or imaginary creatures, griffons and dragons and elephants, their faces often expressing human emotions; or Herbals illustrating herbs in medicinal use. Large numbers of the books were destroyed at the Dissolution of the Monasteries, or cut up and used as paintings ('Cut up missal in evening – hard work' wrote that passionate admirer of medieval art, John Ruskin). The earlier books were produced on parchment by monastic scribes using quills cut from crow or swan feathers, black ink made from the glands of cuttlefish or crushed charcoal or dissolved lamp black. Best of all they liked the more durable iron-gall ink which came from the tumour-like growth around the gall wasp eggs laid in oak trees. They used gold beaten into sheets thinner than tissue, and having ground their pigments they mixed them with a medium of beaten and strained egg-white: the green of malachite, the red and orange of red lead and vermillion (produced by heating mercury and sulphur), the yellow of saffron or arsenic sulphide (how many scribes were poisoned, ending up in the infirmary?); and they used organic pigments: the blue of indigo, the rose of the madder plant, the purple of the turnsole plant. Best of all was ultramarine, its source lapis lazuli, the recipe from 'beyond the sea', from ancient Persia; and for the borders, liquid gold.

They speak of another world, one in which daily life was steeped in the language and imagery of the liturgy; one which reflects a holistic view of man and the harmony of creation; one which sees the whole culture as predominantly Christian with no cut-and-dried distinction between the sacred and the secular. All of it is set against a fearsome background of war, poverty, famine and plague where death was a daily possibility and where life was indeed 'solitary, poor, nasty, brutish and short'. And yet where faith was unchallenged and as natural as breathing. We can't imagine their lives, any more than they could imagine ours. Novelists and historians may come close to reconstructing how they lived and even what they thought, and we may use the same churches and cathedrals and study their writings and their art, but we have little real idea of the impact that faith made on the lives of folk so unlike (and yet so like) us, and who viewed the world as God's domain and the stories of Jesus as a central and familiar part of their lives. Which is why the imagery of these illustrated books, the homeliness of them, still has such power to move us.

We know too much to return to that more innocent world-view. As scientists and theologians uncover new aspects of truth we test such developing knowledge against what we believe. We are beyond them in factual knowledge, though perhaps not in wisdom. Most of us find pretty chilling the scraps that remain of medieval 'Doom' wall-paintings which once instilled the fear of God and his judgement from the walls of village churches, yet their often tiny representations of some of the central truths of the Gospel, captured with such devotion, speak from the heart with potent skill and still convey the eternal truth of the things of God.

10th September

My seventy-sixth birthday. Sarah, Adam and Anna come for lunch and tea. Mentally, still feel all ages at once; physically, though hopefully temporarily, about 105. Never been more aware of the Psalmist's 'The years of our age are three score years and ten, and though men may be so strong that they come to fourscore years, yet is their strength then but labour and sorrow; so soon passeth it away and we are gone.' A. gives me the handsome new *Birds Britannica*; and I eat my birthday cake with difficulty and crumbled in yoghurt.

'Three score years and ten' is no more than a heartbeat in relation to the age of the universe. It is claimed that if you

stand with your arms stretched out to their fullest extent
and imagine that length as the history of the Earth, then the
distance from the fingertips of one hand to the wrist of the
other is the Precambrian era (which ended some 570 million
years ago, and which saw the first fossils and sea urchins).
The whole of the developing, complex life of the universe is
contained in one hand, and 'in a single stroke with a med-
ium-grained nail file you could eradicate human history'.[67] If
we were able to fly backwards into the past at the rate of one
year per second, it would take us about half-an-hour to reach
the time of Christ; three weeks to get to the beginning of
human life; twenty years to reach the dawn of the Cambrian
period.

Thinking *big*, our world is part of one of 140 billion
galaxies that are at present visible to the Mount Hubble
telescope, and if each galaxy was the size of a frozen pea,
there would be enough of them to fill the Royal Albert Hall.
Thinking *small*, we have ten thousand trillion cells in our
bodies, almost each one containing some six feet of densely
packed DNA, each one carrying a copy of our unique genetic
code. Each cell in my body carries the instruction book for
100,000 genes: that's with as many working parts as a Boe-
ing 777. Facts like this may put us in our place, but not so
that we should be overcome by our seeming insignificance,
but rather, that we are able to view the universe and every
cell in our bodies, as awesome, as objects of wonder. Every
part of it finely balanced to create and then support life;
each cell unceasing in its specific task of preserving and
nurturing this old body. And those cells which have rebelled
soon to be zapped by radiation.

11th September: Reflecting on forgiveness, new life
... and death (2)
To the cathedral Eucharist. A visiting preacher with a sermon on personal conversion and what it means to respond
to the forgiveness of God. All good orthodox stuff, but I can
no longer take homilies that are so personalised as to ignore

the implications of that response in terms of the role of the Church as the instrument of the Kingdom, our relationship within the local community or the needs of the world. The termly visit by Godolphin School. An opportunity to say something more relevant to the world they inhabit – not least about the nature of forgiveness in corporate terms. The world is crying out for bread, for clean water, adequate housing, affordable medicine, and for peace. Our personal response to God in the confession of our largely petty failures is necessary, but is it really sufficient? Shouldn't we aim, during the singing by the choir of the *Agnus Dei* to ask Christ to have mercy not just on our wrong-doing but on our failure to care enough, to go the second mile, to bring to mind what happens when 'good men do nothing' – or not enough? ('The good not done, the love not given, time/ Torn off, unused.')[68] The black underclass left to die in New Orleans happens; many avoidable deaths through AIDS in great swathes of Africa and Asia happen; the continuing turmoil in Iraq and starving babies with flies in their nostrils happen; and body parts in the London Underground. Not our fault? That misses the point. If the Church is to help 'redress the balance' then even a silent remembering in the context of the great act of thanksgiving which is the Eucharist witnesses to our desire to be part of the body whose mission it is to do so; and to do so in the 'minute particulars' that are open to us (not least to become more generous) and of which we may become more aware if this daily suffering is in our hearts alongside the gratitude and the wonder.

But what of forgiveness in more personal terms? Along with guilt and anger, there is one area which priests and counsellors are faced with time and again, especially in the case of sudden death. Unresolved grief. Whether or not we believe in God or are persuaded that forgiveness (forgiving without measure because we have been forgiven beyond measure) lies at the heart of the Gospel, it is very hard to live with the knowledge that you can never now fully put right wrongs that you have done, or wrongs done to you, because death has intervened. There is no more time in which to say the word, or hear the word, that would have laid the past to rest. There is a haunting description by George Bernard Shaw of how he stood at the foot of the bed of his dead wife, unable now to speak the words he should have said years before. In George Eliot's *Adam Bede*, Adam reflects on the relationship with his drunken father who has died in an accident:

> Adam's mind rushed back in a flood of relenting and pity. When Death, the Great Reconciler, has come, it is never our tenderness we repent of, but our severity. [Later he learns to think back to what] the old man's feelings had been in moments of humiliation, when he had held down his head before the rebukes of his son, [and wonders how he might act differently given a second chance]. I've known what it is to repent and feel it is too late.[69]

For death, while it is the great leveller, is not in itself the 'Great Reconciler'. If you believe that death is the end, that the singular integrity of this unique combination of body, mind and spirit is now utterly extinguished, then it will be harder to come to terms with that mixture of emptiness, anger and guilt that grief so often brings. 'What might I have done, what might we have said, that we failed ever to say or do? And now it's too late.' One way through this anguish may lie in talking to an experienced bereavement counsellor *for as long as it takes*, and so coming to a fresh understanding of unresolved feelings and find, in time, some healing.

Christians have seen death in a different context, as final as a corpse but less ultimate than the darkness of the grave or just a handful of dust. If you believe that God in Christ is the great Reconciler, that it is this sense of God which explains our lifelong desire for personal integration, that we are embodied spirits with a haunting sense of goodness, still imperfect whenever death strikes, then God is not simply the origin and ground of our deepest experiences of love and forgiveness, beauty and truth. He is their end, their culmination. Our destiny. To hope for heaven is to set our yearning, our hunger for answers that will satisfy our quest for meaning, within the broader context of that new quality of life which the New Testament writers call 'eternal'. A word which doesn't signify unending time – how could it when time has become meaningless? – but life of a different quality. And which they believe begins here and now. In other words, we creatures have chosen to enter into an unbreakable relationship with our Creator which God will honour. 'People who dwell in God', wrote Meister Eckhart, 'dwell in the Eternal Now.' That deepest of mysteries, Incarnation leading to Resurrection, means that Jesus is an ever-present icon, in time yet beyond it, leading us – as all icons seek to do – from a contemplation of the temporal and the visible (his acts of self-sacrificing love) to the enigma of the invisible and the eternal.

We constantly underestimate the power of God to create and re-create. At certain critical points in the process of evolution new forms of life have emerged, each with new potential, as infinitely slowly the true nature of the Creator-spirit is discerned, until in the person of Jesus something quite new occurs. Easter speaks of God inaugurating *a new stage in creation*, for in this definitive life and death our own life and death are redefined. God reveals in Jesus the kind of human life which can become fully life with God, not only here and now, but eternally beyond the threshold of death. So we stand with Edwin Muir's 'one foot in Eden', one foot in time and one foot in eternity, for it is in the risen Christ that we catch the scent of what God is and what we are created to be.

So if you believe that death is not our ultimate destiny, then the possibility of forgiving and receiving forgiveness from those whom we love but no longer see takes on a new meaning. For you both still lie within that enfolding relationship with God which exists either side of death. Not in the sense of Scott Holland's less-than-helpful phrase so popular at memorial services, 'I'm only in the next room', which trivialises the awesome reality of death. But, more profoundly, in the belief that in Christ love for the invisible loved one (and so mutual forgiveness) may still be given and received, a necessary part of the leave-taking.

Other deaths are more drawn out. When cancer is diagnosed, that is not in itself a death sentence. Many cancers can be cured; others put in abeyance through drugs or other treatments. But it is a tap on the shoulder, a healthy (or unhealthy) reminder of your mortality. The kaleidoscope of your life shifts a little. And it focuses the mind on how we should prepare for that inevitable close. Unlike a sudden fatal heart attack, stroke or terminal accident, or even the slow descent into senility, cancer allows us time, be it months or years, to order our affairs and say what needs to be said. My greatly valued friend Cicely Saunders, whose vision of the modern hospice changed our whole approach to dying and to enabling people to live well until the end, told me years ago that she would like to die of cancer in the hospice she founded. A week before my operation we spoke on the phone and said goodbye. She was dying of cancer at St Christopher's. A few days later she died very peacefully. 'Say a prayer for me when you get there,' I said. 'Oh, I will.' Though where 'there' may be, of course, neither of us had the least idea.

12th September

My Shopmobility scooter again. No time to write: England win the Ashes.

13th September

Another lovely early autumn day. Pick blackberries at Hurdcott. Coffee at the local pub. Swallows still here. The fields full of stubble. It was on 21 September 1819 that John Keats wrote to his friend J. H. Reynolds:

How beautiful the season is now – how fine the air ... I never
liked stubble fields so much as now, ay, better than the chilly
green of the spring. Somehow a stubble plain looks warm – in
the same way that some pictures look warm. This struck me so
much in my Sunday's walk that I composed upon it.[70]

What he composed was the 'Ode to Autumn'.

Watch the wonderfully escapist *Pirates of the Caribbean*,
though A. prefers to read Julian Barnes.

14th September

Four appointments booked for Southampton Hospital next
week, including a CT scan and the moulding of the radiotherapy mask, so they're moving reasonably fast. Mouth still
very swollen and sore, and swellings in neck and throat
unchanged in a month. Less discomfort from heavy bruising
on leg and shoulder. Face still numb. It will be eight weeks
on Friday.

15th September

To Salisbury Playhouse for matinée of fine production of
Harper Lee's *To Kill a Mockingbird*. Placed firmly in the
wheelchair box.

16th September: Reflecting on words (3)

Sometimes I feel overwhelmed by the sheer weight of books
demanding attention and the shortness of time ahead. 'Look
at me!' they clamour from the loaded shelves of novels,
biographies, essays, poetry, short stories, some still unread
after possessing them for half a lifetime. (And, up in my
study, some much-weeded shelves containing some well-
tested theology.) Many more books plead, 'Look at me
again!' They challenge the steady trickle of new books whose
claim seems equally valid. I have learned much more about
human nature – and, I believe, about the transcendent,
about good and evil, sin and grace – from the novelist and
the poet than from the theologian, where only rare writers

THE QUESTIONING COUNTRY OF CANCER

combine the insight, the humanity and the sheer readability that draw you back to them. The greatest novels – *Madame Bovary*, *War and Peace*, *Anna Karenina*, *Pride and Prejudice*, *Middlemarch*, *Crime and Punishment*, *Tess* and *Jude* and *Bleak House* – are not didactic: in their universality they show life in all its messiness, their characters allowed to make moral choices which may or may not be the author's, and shaped by those choices for good or ill. They show us, too, that the choices the characters make have the inevitable effect of touching and changing, enhancing or damaging, the lives of others. Milan Kundera, the Czech novelist, writes of *Anna Karenina* that it is 'the imaginary paradise where no one possesses the truth, neither Anna nor Karenin, but where everyone has the right to be understood, both Anna and Karenin'.[71] 'Where everyone has the right to be understood': that's what impels the creative imagination of the writer and the empathetic response of the reader. The possibility, through a listening that is not judgemental, of getting inside another's skin, the enlarging of your own understanding of what it is to be someone else. We respond to certain books, plays and films, not just because they say something authentic about our own lives, but because they can awaken an awareness of other realities, other personalities, other people's lives.

> When I let myself be affected by a book, [writes Jeanette Winterson] I let myself into new customs and new desires. The book does not reproduce me, it redefines me, pushes at my boundaries, shatters the palings that guard my heart. Strong texts work along the borders of our minds and alter what already exists.[72]

(Winterson was brought up in a strict Brethren household where only six books were permitted: two Bibles, Cruden's *Concordance for the Old and New Testaments*, *The Chatterbox Annual 1923* and *The House at Pooh Corner*. She discovered that 77 paperbacks are the maximum number you can hide under an average single-bed mattress without a suspicious rise in its level.)

No one has written better about the power and limitation of words than George Steiner. He believes that the words of the poet or the philosopher will always fall short of 'the numinous intensities of certain phenomena and states of felt being'. In other words, some human experiences, especially that of 'the otherness of things', the impenetrable nature of certain aspects of life, the underlying mystery of why there is anything at all, face us with the question of why, if this is a Godless universe with everything explicable in terms of evolution dictated by 'the selfish gene', there should be art and poetry and music. Steiner speaks of the experience we may have of entering into a deeply personal relationship with a poem, a painting, a piece of music which is an undeniable part of our humanness yet impossible to describe to anyone else; of how it seems 'to call on us ... the process of penetration, of implantation [suggesting] a chemical bonding'.[73] Ultimately, words fail. They give way to silence. Music and silence. We can only say: 'It is; we are.'

17th September: Reflecting on words (4)

Reading *Snow* by Orhan Pamuk, an outstanding novelist brave enough to write freely of Turkey's place in the modern world. Earlier this year, in a Swiss newpaper, Panuk asserted that 'a million Armenians and 30,000 Kurds were killed (in the alleged Armenian Massacre of 1915), and no one dares to talk about it except me'. There was an immediate call for his books to be burned, and he awaits trial for 'denigrating Turkey', a charge that carries a three-year jail sentence, in December. (*Later:* after appearing in court and being jeered and manhandled, the charges against him were dropped.)

We stand in a tradition in which the primacy of the word was carried over from Greek and Judaic cultures into the Christian tradition, one in which words sought to contain the sum of human experience; in which it was the Word that was made flesh and spoke words which have burrowed deep into the human psyche. It has been esimated that our language contains some 600,000 words (though how many are in use is another question). Some 150,000 words were available to Shakespeare; those who translated the King James version of the Bible made do with just 6000. Why do words matter so much? Why, for some, do books become a passion, even an obsession? Though for how much longer? Computer technology and the net have changed the way human beings communicate and (at their best) open up new possibilities for education in the Third World. And (at their worst) swamp the world with quirky blogs and unwanted, lubricious e-mails. Microchips have transformed the music business, DVDs have done the same for the film industry, books can be read off a computer; and it is almost certainly only a matter of time before someone patents a portable electronic reader that looks like paper and which allows books to be downloaded onto it straight from the internet. And yet ... more books are published than ever before and the quality of the best of them shows no sign of diminishing. In the past year 161,000 new titles have been published in the United Kingdom, and last year 296 million books were sold. Book clubs are mushrooming everywhere, what Robert McCrum calls 'middle England's bingo'.

Different kinds of writing convey different ways of communicating truth. Even the most scholarly of historians and the most conscientious of biographers can only hope to illuminate aspects of a life. People tend to think that the meaning of 'fiction' is 'I make things up as I go along'. But it isn't. Aristotle in his *Poetics* wrote that fiction is 'truer and more universal than history'. 'Fiction' comes from a Latin verb meaning 'I give shape to things', and what the best novelists, poets and playwrights have always done is not only to seek to render the visible world and the desires of the human heart in accurate, authentic words, but to take the untidy human journey and discover a meaning in it, give it a shape, turn it into fiction in the true sense of the word. Ideas, reflections, observations, from different ages all

173

preserved like flies in amber. A novelist who deserves to be much better known is Andrei Makine. He was born in Siberia, from where he escaped to Paris, seeking asylum there, living rough and writing as he sat on park benches. He has written nine novels and won several literary prizes. In one of the best of them, *Le Testament Francais*, a mixture of autobiography and fiction, he writes of his magical discovery of words:

> Literature was now revealed as being perpetual amazement at the flow of words into which the world dissolved ... True literature was that magic, a word, a verse, a chapter of which transported us into a changeless moment of beauty.[74]

Words used to convey 'perpetual amazement': time and again in his novels he captures the sense of the significance, the timelessness, of ordinary moments.

Aristotle wrote that the main purpose of tragedy was to awaken pity and terror, together with a sense of awe at our potential, not simply to bear and not be overcome by suffering, but to redeem it, to bring something good out of a dark time. He saw it as an assertion of human value in the face of what so often seems a hostile universe. Neither words nor music can of themselves prevent the terror that repression brings, but during the siege of Sarajevo Vedran Smailovi played his cello in the rubble-strewn streets and lifted people's spirits; and a performance of Beckett's *Waiting for Godot* actually helped lift the siege. Sometimes the words fail, and music falls silent, in the face of iconic visual images – the figure dying on the Cross; the young man facing alone the tanks in Tiananmen Square; the starving child in Darfur. Yet words can find striking, universal images to render the horror of war or the wonder of first love; equally they can witness to truth in a tyranny or be twisted to suit the purposes of a corrupt regime. Seamus Heaney has written of how poetry (and it is no less true of novels and plays) 'encompasses the desolations of reality, and remains, like hope, an indispensible part of being human'. He sees poetry as being pitched between things as they are and things as they should be. He has written, in a series of essays now collected as *Finders Keepers*, of dissident poets like Zbigniew Herbert who guaranteed in war-time and post-war Communist Poland the survival of the valid self and of the good and the beautiful, 'or rather ... the responsibility of each person to ensure that survival',[75] one who writes that

> we look in the face of hunger the face of fire the face of death
> worst of all – the face of betrayal
> and only our dreams have not been humiliated.[76]

He writes of the great Czeslaw Milosz, witness to the Warsaw Ghetto uprising and its defeat by the Nazis, whose work combines lyrical beauty and a passionate condemnation of the desolation of the human spirit brought about by Fascism and Marxism. In Heaney's words, 'He will never renege on his glimpses of heaven upon earth, nor on his knowledge that the world is a vale of tears.'[77]

Heaney writes, too, of the poet Joseph Brodsky, the Russian dissident who was arrested in the 1960s by the Soviet authorities and banished to a work-camp in Archangel. He escaped to America, and never ceased to write about the power of poetry as a force for good even in Stalin's Russia. (Brodsky knew how even in the democratic West, as we know to our cost, political systems and the desire to sell newspapers almost inevitably lead to a debasement of language and so to a lowering of what he called 'the plane of regard' from which we view ourselves and establish our values. It's not just in advertising that words are prostituted, chosen for their seductiveness rather than their truthfulness.) In Russia, Brodsky was not alone. As early as 1922, if the arts were to survive at all, artists had to collaborate with the Bolshevik regime. Stalin set up a directorate and undesirable works, native or foreign, were banned. Before long all written works submitted to publishers had also to be submitted to the Politburo. A few writers protested: others, like Gorky, fell into line. Among the brave few were Osip

Mandelstam and Anna Akhmatova (and, some decades later, Solzhenitsyn and Irina Ratushinskaya, the former with his courageous, powerful novels, the latter exiled and imprisoned in Siberia, from where she smuggled out her poems on tiny scraps of paper). Mandelstam was forced to abandon poetry, given ten years' hard labour, and sent to Siberia, where the first harsh winter killed him. After 1932, poetry critical of the regime had to be committed to memory, and such punishable views only surfaced in the folk-songs of those in the camps or herded together on collective farms. At the same time, the censors and party officials removed half the books from public libraries and publishing came under the control of the Central Committee. Donald Rayfield, in his book *Stalin and His Hangmen*,[78] writes that 'music not in C Major, poetry that was not paraphrasable, painting and film not monumental or strictly representational, were all banned'. But censorship may be self-imposed. As the poet Wallace Stevens wrote:

> No politician can control the imagination, directing it to do this or that. Stalin might grind his teeth the whole of a Russian winter and yet all the poets in the Soviets might remain silent the following spring.[79]

More recently, the Czech writer Vaclav Havel, who ran the unlikely gamut from imprisoned dissident to President of the Republic, claimed that every cultural act was 'good in and of itself, because it exists and because it offers something to someone ... even if only for a moment, perhaps to a single person', and that this somehow changes the state of things, the common good, for the better.[80]

Words are powerful tools and can be lethal. Dictators fear them and seek to censor them. But even in democracies there is a different, more subtle, form of silencing at work. In a radio discussion between Joseph Brodsky and George Steiner, Steiner was extolling the supreme value of artistic masterpieces. 'Yes,' said Brodsky, 'but the greatest masterpiece is freedom.' Words play a central part in preserving it.

For freedom implies listening as well as speaking, allowing the voiceless to find a voice. Britain is not excluded from the nations in which many are denied a voice: women, children, the old and powerless, asylum-seekers, those producing cheap goods for world markets in the world's sweatshops, prisoners of conscience, those denied a trial in our own detention centres or in Guantanamo Bay. When we fail to listen or deny them language we deny their humanity. Abuse flourishes where the words end, where voices of protest or despair are silenced, whether through racial harassment (Jews during the Third Reich, Palestinians driven from their homelands), casual or deliberate neglect, or violence. Different cultures use different methods, from the burning of books to the literal cutting out of tongues. Words can be twisted to justify anything, even torture.

In Britain, fear over terrorist activities has brought a new sensitivity to the question of freedom of expression in which politicians and public are by no means of one mind. From Socrates to the Magna Carta, through Erasmus, John Milton, the Bill of Rights, Voltaire and John Stuart Mill, to the UN Declaration of Human Rights, the right to free speech has been sacrosanct to any democratic nation. But the new reality of worldwide terrorism and the rise of religious extremism have brought about a new debate concerning the threatening use of language about what others hold sacred. This means that this enshrined liberty must be set against the right to be protected against the violence of gratuitous offence. And that's where the tough decisions begin. An essential tolerance is severely tested when extremists disgorge their views in hurtful and offensive language. We live now in a deeply secular state. It's hard to defend the kind of blinkered secularism which pours scorn on those they consider feeble-minded for still affirming Christian belief. For that equally devalues people by denying the validity of what they most deeply believe and seek to live by. The fact that it's done in the most civilised of ways shouldn't disguise the fact that it is akin to the extremism we jointly condemn.

Writ small, but of the same genus. Whatever the outcome of the current debate about the restriction of liberty, one of the least attractive aspects of our national life is the practice in parts of the tabloid press of marginalising people as 'stranger', 'enemy', 'outsider', the ones who have no rights and who don't belong. To remain silent in the face of such crude labelling is to connive with the desire to silence those whose words no longer count. It contains ominous echoes of the repressive regimes of the twentieth century. And, like radiation, it is cumulative in its effects.

Yet words properly valued are among our most precious gifts, not least those used by writers to point to the wonder and mystery of the creation and to our inborn sense of beauty, desire and compassion, and our common experience of suffering. Like the great belief systems, they tell us how we stumble and fall, and how we can survive and stand tall again. Just as Christianity is not about providing neat answers to life's problems (though some preachers speak as if it were, using words as if they were hard metal rather than air), but about encountering mystery, so birth and death and all that lies between are not meant to be explained but experienced and described in words that will make our living and dying important again. The American poet Stanley Kunitz came to believe that the most wonderful thing (to write about) is 'the mystery and beauty of ordinary human existence'. He believed words to be so erotic, 'they never tire of their coupling. How do they renew themselves? In their inexhaustible desire for combinations and recombinations.'[81]

But they must come from the heart. As Beethoven wrote on the manuscript of his *String Quartet No 16 in F Major*: 'From the heart: it must go to the heart.' (Steiner laments the dying-out of learning poetry *by heart*, 'a term beautifully apposite to the organic inward presentation of meaning and spoken being within the individual spirit'.)[82] The Word of God, speaking all things into being through the miracle of freely evolving life, is heard with new and startling force

178

when it is made flesh in one whose words and actions, and whose stories about their familiar world, persuaded those who heard them that they came from the heart, not just of this man, but of his Father. ('He who has seen me has seen the Father.') As Muriel Bradbrook used to say: 'the beating heart of the universe now beating beneath a human heart'. Equally, if our words are to speak with authenticity (and authority), they must be rooted, incarnated, in our familiar world, the world of the lover, the parent, the child; of the workplace and the cancer ward.

'Poetry', writes R. S. Thomas, 'is that which arrives at the intellect/ By way of the heart.'[83] Every serious writer seeks to speak from the heart of what rings true of the world about them and about the mingled yarn of their lives. Some believe in God; many don't. Some are persuaded that when God says in effect, 'I give you my word' in Jesus Christ, we find in that life of selfless love the essence of the Being who is to be trusted and who holds all things in being. But the discovery of truth is not limited to theologians or scientists, and at their most persuasive the poet's words, the novelist's words, the playwright's words – or the artist's image, the sculptor's carving, the composer's manuscript – may help to authenticate the inner promptings of our spirits. The best of them help to confirm what we too have experienced but did not till then have the words for, though as soon as they are in print – or on the canvas, emerging from the wood or stone, or being performed – we claim them as our own. For they speak of what 'human' feels like, and we can say, 'Yes, that's how it is for me too.'

The octogenarian Bishop John Cavell visits me. Before he goes I ask him to bless me. He replies, 'No, I want *you* to bless *me.*' A perceptive and thoughtful act, affirming my priesthood in the only way possible at present.

18th September: Reflecting on art ... and incarnation

Yesterday I wrote of the power of words, and even more of music, to speak to the heart, and of how in the Incarnation God addresses the heart in the most powerful way he could. But what of art? Art whose purpose is to trap the passing moment and capture the feelings we may share when we experience life most intensely. Art which can discern the harmony under the tangle of existence, the seeming chaos, and make visible to us the beauty of rhythm, line, shape, structure, colour, hinting at a longed-for perfection which reflects the infinite beauty of God. ('The beauty of being', wrote Spinoza, 'is the real name for God.') Certain paintings and sculpture, poems, music – Bellini's *Holy Family*, Michelangelo's *Pieta*, a Keats Ode, Bach's *Goldberg Variations* (make your own choice) – may have a deeply satisfying inevitability so that it's hard to imagine they could be other than they are.

> *Incarnation: n.* Embodiment in (esp. human) flesh, esp. the Incarnation (of Christ); impersonation, living type (of quality etc.); (M.E. f. eccl. Lat. *incarnatio*).

Not all that helpful. When we speak of 'incarnation', we sometimes mean '*the* Incarnation', that bridge between God and us: a unique enfleshing, the embodiment in a human life of that beauty, goodness and truth which are intrinsic to and mirror the being of God. It is about making the infinite finite, revealing the eternal in time, spirit in matter; truths humans could only guess at displayed in visible, tactile flesh. But the concept of 'incarnation' has a far wider import than the Word once made flesh, for incarnation is a principle of all creation and we need to see the imprint of God everywhere in our universe, the Creator's mind and spirit undergirding the whole wondrous process of evolution, and sustaining his work moment by moment. Such a concept looks for the spiritual in and through the everyday: it sanctifies the ordinary. So Ruskin saw the stones and trees on simple hillsides as 'incarnations' of God's activity. Constable and Turner and English watercolourists in particular seemed to him to capture the most fugitive and beautiful of natural phenomena in which he felt he could perceive the divine presence – as opposed to Dutch art, of which he had a low view, describing it as 'the patient devotion of besotted lives to the delineation of bricks and fogs, cattle and ditchwater'. Franz Hals? Rembrandt? And can the way Vermeer and De Hooch transform those ordinary interiors and brick couryards into something memorable and extraordinary merely be decribed as 'patient devotion', lacking the divine presence?

Plato wrote of beauty in terms of his belief that the world of visible matter is but a reflection of the real but invisible world. For him, the real world is that of ideas and of the Ideal, and everything that exists has its corresponding form in the world of ideas, the Ideal, as it were, imprinting its pattern upon matter. Plotinus, following Plato, explains our yearning for the beautiful by distinguishing between beauty in the natural world, the human face and body, and the greater beauty of character, the innocence of young children for example, what we might call 'moral' beauty, both of which attract us. He thought of each person as a dual entity, each soul as trapped by matter but as a fragment of the Divine Being with a longing to be restored. So Wordsworth famously wrote in 'Intimations of Immortality from Reflections of early Childhood':

> Not in entire forgetfulness,
> And not in utter nakedness,
> But trailing clouds of glory do we come
> From God, who is our home.

What links art and spirituality is the sense of wonder, and when we encounter what to us is beautiful, recognise it as such and respond with gratitude for such an unexpected gift, we are exercising what seems a uniquely human gift. And 'this thrill, this sense of recognition, is what we call "the experience of beauty'".[84] When artists convey a sense of beauty they are therefore giving us an experience of perfection, harmony and order which are the qualities that the soul is striving for, not imposing anything we don't already possess, but seeking to stir the memory of that which already exists within us. So one main function of art is to incarnate truth and beauty, to define 'human', to tell us who we truly are. Many artists, of course, convey quite different emotions, for art also has a provocative role. It should hold a mirror up to the world, and what we see may sometimes disturb or disgust us. Picasso's *Guernica* or Goya's *Horrors of War* stir our sense of pity and compassion, equally beautiful when given voice and acted upon. For Picasso, the object of art was always 'to shock into recognition'.

At its best, art, no less than religion, is about the need to search for the reality behind the everyday, even if much modern art seems an expression of our estrangement from nature and the futility of human existence. P. T. Forsyth, writing on art and religion at the start of the twentieth century, believed that the weakness of British art at that time was due to what he called our weak 'Anglo-Saxon Theism, imperfectly Christianised as yet by the principle of Incarnation'. He regretted the loss of a theology

> which is not only tolerated by the public intelligence, but is welcome for the life, commanding for the reason, and fascinating for the imagination of the age ... a faith that represents the Divine man rather than the human God.[85]

In other words, a faith with a deep sense of the immanence of God within his world. Not just in 'the Word made flesh', nor in terms of pantheism, which would too easily identify God with the creation, but the belief that God combines both transcendence and immanence: in other words, that it is pervaded and held in being by his creative Spirit, that he indwells it, rather as (though all analogies are inadequate) my 'self' permeates my body yet transcends it and can't be identified with any one part of it. The God who is within as well as the God who is beyond: mysterious yet available, unimaginable yet incarnate, the divine paradox with which we shall continue to wrestle all our days. Even if my computer-thesaurus spell-check stubbornly sticks to pantheism, *The Oxford Dictionary of the Christian Church* also embraces *panentheism*, which is the belief that 'the Being of God includes and penetrates the whole universe, so that every part of it exists in Him, but (as against *pantheism*) that His Being is more than, and is not exhausted by, the universe'. Augustine confessed to God that 'the beautiful things of the world kept me far from you and yet, if they had not been in you, they would have had no being at all'.[86] John V. Taylor always insisted that the religious experience of the numinous and the aesthetic experience of the beautiful only differed in degree, not in kind, that certain kinds of aesthetic perception were as valid, and no less an experience of transcendence, than more mystical or numinous ones. Each offers 'an insight into the nature of that "otherness" that is common to them all'.[87] Just as God in the Incarnation identifies himself with the ordinariness of human life, so we come to see that nothing is merely 'ordinary', for all is extraordinary once we come to see *into* it with eyes of perception. We become blinded by matter, failing to see through to the spirit that informs it. Charles Gore wrote of the doctrine of the Holy Spirit as that 'wherein God touches man most nearly, most familiarly, in common life'. An interesting, if minor, English artist, Winifred Nicholson, painted a delicate study of a small pot of lilies-of-the-valley, and said that the flowers 'held the secret of the universe'. ('To see the world in a grain of sand/ And heaven in a wild flower . . .')

The last recorded words of Poussin were: 'Painting is an imitation in lines and colours of all that is under the sun.' And so it is. It is the attempt to capture on canvas all that is contained in one transient moment and what may lie beneath that moment which gives it a feel of eternity. Every serious artist searches for self-transcendence, some in the belief that there are absolute values. Many have what Evelyn Underhill called 'an intuition of the Real lying at the root of the visible world and sustaining its life'.[88] The creation is in constant flux, and the landscape painter takes on this ceaseless movement, or the still-life painter seeks to arrest the constant dispersal of objects, and they stop us in our tracks, inviting us to look at life and love it at this or that captured instant, the subject in a state of absolute rest. But how on earth do you capture the light and shadow that never stand still but are always changing? That was the great challenge faced by the Impressionists, and Monet tries to resolve it by painting his haystacks and line of poplars and Rouen Cathedral in all their moods in the shifting light. The Impressionists speak so powerfully because they sought to convey in the familiar and the everyday a lost spiritual dimension. Cézanne called painting 'a coloured state of grace', and described nature as 'the spectacle that the *Pater Omnipotens* and *Aeternae Deus* spreads out before our eyes'; his desire was to restore to objects their true radiance. Renoir sought to capture what he called 'that state of grace which comes from contemplating God's most beautiful creation, the human body'; van Gogh, who saw the natural world as seething with divine life, wrote of how he wanted to paint men and women 'with that something of the eternal which the halo used to symbolise, but which we now seek to counter through the actual radiance of colour vibrations'; and, a little later, Matisse said that it was the human figure that 'fills me with awe towards life'. The painter Paul Nash turned to landscape painting not 'for the landscape's sake but for the "things behind", the dweller in the innermost: whose light shines thro' sometimes';[89] and the sculptor Barbara Hepworth wrote that in the contemplation of nature (where we find 'the greatest and purest sculptural process of all, the action of the universe on the surface of the earth')

we are perpetually renewed, our sense of mystery and imagination are kept alive, and if rightly understood, it gives us the power to project into a plastic medium some universal and abstract vision of beauty.[90]

Contemplating art, giving our absorbed attention to a painting or sculpture that speaks to us and demands a response, is one of the few ways given to us to relate to that parallel dimension which, for want of a better word, we call 'eternity'.

One of the most interesting changes of heart has been in the strongly materialist art critic and former Marxist, John Berger. By the mid-1980s he was writing of 'the phenomenon of grace'; and in *The White Bird* he writes:

> Art is an organised response to what nature allows us to glimpse occasionally. Art sets out to transform the potential recognition into an unceasing one. It proclaims man in the hope of receiving a surer reply ... The transcendental face of art is always a form of prayer.[91]

Interesting, too, is the response of George Steiner. In his *Real Presences* he writes:

> Where we read truly, where the experience is to be that of meaning, we do so as if the text (the piece of music, the work of art) *incarnates ... a real presence of significant being ... To be indwelt by music, art, literature ... is to experience the commonplace mystery of a real presence.*[92] [My italics.]

No doubt it's the *nature* of that presence on which we should disagree.

Sometimes pictures speak when words are silenced. Two days after the destruction of New York's Twin Towers on 9/11 I was at a hospice conference. At the final session we were supposed to talk about what it had achieved. But still stunned by that act of terrorism we asked instead for a huge roll of paper, and armed with paint and crayons we all knelt round silently on the floor and produced a great collage of images that expressed our emotions much better than any words we might have found.

185

Above all, perhaps, the arts give us delight. They can speak to our need for times of play as well as times of work, of our need to be fed by passion and beauty and laughter and hope. It is said that one day Goethe was told that Haydn in his old age had been asked why his masses were so gay and not at all ceremonious and solemn: to which Haydn replied, 'When I think of the good God I am filled with gaiety.' Upon which Goethe burst into tears.

19th September

To Southampton General Hospital. A demanding morning. Session with consultant, C.B. Then strip off and lie flat and still for the simulator to line me up and for the lasers to show where the radiation will be centered: a wide triangle from the left ear to the breastbone and across the mouth and throat to a point on the right side of the chin, the lines marked with red and black pens in an ominous tattoo. A metal prong attached to a ball of plastic is inserted in my mouth to allow me to breathe (and, during radiation, to help protect the top side of the tongue, even if, as it proved, pretty ineffectively). Then on to the moulding room. Strip again and lie flat: to guarantee stillness they strap me down. Again lined up with lasers. Then my neck, face, shoulders and chest are coated with vaseline, my hair bound in clingfilm. A thick pink sludge is then quickly spread on the whole of my top half, covering (help!) eyes and ears and nose, leaving just the nostrils free. White plaster is then slapped on top of the pink mixture, and slowly hardens. It feels hot, heavy and oppressive, a bit claustrophobic, as if you're being mummified or prepared for some ancient burial rite. After six minutes the whole is cut and violently stripped away, taking most of the chest hairs with it. It all takes 40 minutes, and from it they will make my individual mould. Not an experience I'd want every day.

20th September

Oral Clinic at 9. See I.D. He confirms a persistent lump in the roof of my mouth is not cancerous. Guess that this is how it will be from now on if suspicious swellings appear. Story in today's paper of the latest smash-hit in the States, *The March of the Penguins*, a documentary claiming that Emperor penguins in the Antarctic go through horrendous conditions in their devoted rearing of their young. Claimed by the American religious right as affirming God's intelligent design, illustrating the traditional values of monogamy, selflessness and faithful child-rearing; moreover the crude act of mating is not shown. Tests carried out at Bremen Zoo earlier this year, however, showed that out of five pairings studied, three pairs turned out to be gay. Nor do most Emperor penguins mate for life. Darwinians ten: Creationists nil.

This is a strange, in-between sort of time. Feel better than I have for the past year, with more energy (though not *much* more). Yet I know that October/November will be challenging with the radiotherapy centring on that most sensitive area, the mouth. I am savouring every taste at present in case, as they warn, the tastebuds are destroyed rather than temporarily stunned. If so, what tastes shall I miss most? Raspberries, bitter chocolate, Glastonbury cheese, Cox's Orange pippins, the first broad beans, coffee and draught bitter. And least? Beetroot.

21st September: Reflecting on prayer (2) and the *cantus firmus*

There's a story of a man attending a boxing match knowing nothing of the rules of boxing. A friend explains them to him. As the boxers climb into the ring, one crosses himself. 'What does that mean?' he asks. 'It don't mean a thing if he can't box,' replies the friend. Sometimes when we try to pray or join together in worship, although we go through all the right motions, we find that we're pretty hopeless at both. Those who conduct services are inevitably concerned with the performance of the liturgy, that it may be so ordered as to give others the best chance of an experience (however fleeting) both of the numinous and of their membership of a worshipping body. Perhaps only in retirement do those forced to function at the sharp end, in pulpits or in prayer stalls or behind altars, have the chance to relax and give their unselfconscious attention to what they are doing, seeking to be receptive to the Spirit. But that's hard too. For it's part of being human that whenever we turn aside to worship or to pray (alone or with others) all kinds of frustrating things start to happen. Last Sunday I listened to the first part of a sermon which was so stimulating that my mind took off along a parallel track – and missed the punchline. During the intercessions I began thinking of Iraqi civilians when others had fast-forwarded to prayers for the departed. At home this morning, as so often, I began to say my prayers and quickly began to drift into a seamless stream of consciousness.

> I throwe myselfe downe in my Chamber, [said John Donne with characteristic honesty] and I call God in, and invite God and his Angels thither, and when they are there, I neglect God and his Angels, for the noise of a Flie, for the ratling of a Coach, for the whining of a Doore; I talk on … Eyes lifted up; knees bowed downe; as though I prayed to God; and if God or his Angels should aske me, when I last thought of God in that prayer, I cannot tell … A memory of yesterday's pleasures, a feare of tomorrow's dangers, a straw under my knee, a noise in mine eare, a light in mine eye, an any thing, a nothing, a fancy … troubles me in my prayer. So certainly there is nothing … in spirituall things perfect in this world.[93]

Sometimes you can turn these unsought-for thoughts into prayer, but it's all a bit messy and undisciplined, and leaves us feeling that we may be going through all the right motions 'but it don't mean a thing' if we can't still our minds for long enough to give God a chance to speak. In the words of Claudius: 'My words fly up, my thoughts remain below,/ Words without thoughts never to heaven go.'

And yet ... (as I wrote in Part I) this is where I turn again to my belief in the *cantus firmus*: a foundation laid down over the years, and made up of those moments in common worship (brief epiphanies, Virginia Woolf's 'candles lit in the dark') when I have strongly sensed the hidden, lurking presence of my Creator. Made up, too, of those rare times when praying or reading alone, and something more of the truths implicit in the words 'Incarnation', 'Cross' and 'Eucharist' and a God who is Christlike has struck fire within me and endorsed the firm ground at my centre. So that when I feel nothing during an act of worship, or when my mind takes off during prayer, I say to God:

> Loving Father, Source and End of my life, you know me infinitely better than I shall ever know myself; there is within me that which lies deeper than these trivial and inadequate words and random thoughts. Do not simply look on what I am but on what in my heart I desire to be.

Or words to that effect.

Go to a matinée of the new film of *Pride and Prejudice*, surrounded by elderly women who feel free to comment from time to time and are noisily moved at the happy outcome.

22nd–23rd September: Reflection on death (3)

To Southampton for second fitting of the mask. Again head and shoulders totally encased, the plastic wedge in my mouth. They fasten the mask firmly to the table on which I'm lying and use a bunsen-burner to create holes for my ears. Very noisy and strange. Think again of Keats' words: 'nothing is real until it is experienced'. Then a CT scan wearing the mask, injected with a coloured liquid, inserted into the humming machine, tattooed on the chest to mark the point which will guide the radiographers. Another experience I would gladly have missed.

Rabbi John Rayner, one of the leaders of Reform Judaism in Britain and always one of the most welcome of participants at the Abbey's annual Commonwealth Observance, has died. His obituarist records how, writing at the end of his life about being old, Rayner said, 'Although, like Woody Allen, we should still "prefer not to be there when it happens", we become accustomed to our mortality and are less afraid of dying.' I've touched on the subject of death two or three times, but skirted round the related but separate issue of dying. Six months ago, to the question 'Are you afraid?', my answer might have been, 'I don't think so', or on good days, 'No'. But now I'm not so sure, for there's a sense in which we are human before we are Christian and the very human bit retains that primal fear of the dark, the unknown, the 'here lie dragons' of childhood. I suspect a more honest answer would be a very human 'Yes'. What has changed? Two things: the reality of cancer at work, mole-like in your body, bringing with it a new sense of your mortality and a certainty that this is the way you'll go eventually, rather than through a sudden stroke or heart attack. And secondly, a lively memory of the post-operative days when I was 'not myself': hallucinating and irrational and, alone in the small hours, very scared. Suddenly glimpsing what it might feel like to lose control of the power to think clearly or know that your faith is strong enough to face down your fears.

Scared, too, of pain? That as well, though thankfully we live at a time of increasing expertise in palliative care, one that seeks to ensure pain control of a quality previous generations would have envied. I've already written about aspects of 'soul pain', the anguish of leaving those you love and all the familiar scenes that captivate us by their beauty. That, too, will be part of it. But it's knowing that our death is inevitable yet not knowing exactly what form it will take; it's the unpredictability inflamed by an over-active imagination, that makes human beings unique in anticipating and reflecting on how they will face their end.

So what difference does it make to embrace a faith rooted in Jesus Christ and the God he revealed? Can the 'perfect love' (implying absolute trust) of which the First Letter of John speaks, *really* 'cast out fear'? This, surely, is the ultimate test of the *cantus firmus*, of what most deeply motivates our lives. For many people, death remains 'the great unmentionable', yet in the end, for most of us, it proves a peaceful letting-go. And afterwards we shall either be extinguished like a blown-out candle flame and know nothing more, or we shall continue to exist in that ongoing relationship with our Creator in which death is but the sloughing-off of the earthly body which has served us so expertly but is now worn out. Most of my life (and faith is always balanced finely between doubt and confidence) I have believed the latter to be true, not just with my reason but as a truth I feel on my pulse and sense intuitively at the still centre of my being. Life at its finest and best cannot simply be an accidental nonsense. But *dying*, when it means a slow leave-taking, when body and mind are failing, placing an intolerable burden on those who love you, that's what we fear. Yet having the chance to prepare for death, particularly with those you love most, can help them afterwards in the long process of grieving.

I don't believe we are meant to think about what 'human' means (or 'life' or 'death') except in the context of God as their source and culmination, any more than I believe that we are meant to think of God or heaven or the Kingdom except in the context of Jesus Christ. To be a Christian is to learn to see everything through the prism of Christ: to see yourself, and everyone else, to see the world in all its mysterious splendour, and to see the purpose and meaning of your life, newly defined in him. I've spoken of Hugh's phrase, 'the Kingdom-heart', in terms of community and social justice, the readiness to forgive, and in that compassionate concern for the poor and vulnerable which is so deeply ingrained in the Bible. I've written, too, of how we may be motivated to embrace the Pauline trio of 'faith, hope and love', by the conviction that each of us is 'enfolded in Love', that 'nothing can separate us from the love of God in Jesus Christ our Lord'. Not the slow descent into old age, not cancer or Parkinson's or Alzheimer's, nor the agony of grief. It isn't that God steps in to protect us from such assaults. Our bodies must wear out in due course and we must die of *something*. The test lies in how we respond. It may be, for some, with despair. It may be with the Stoic courage, expecting nothing more, of the atheist. Or it may be with the conviction that in death as in life you have been held and sustained by One who has invited your trust and, in Jesus, demonstrated the Love which is at once the most powerful force in creation, both in time and in eternity. Mere words? Maybe; but what else have we with which to clothe and in which to communicate our inmost thoughts? Thoughts about how it may be to die – suddenly in the blink of an eye, or with a gradual withdrawal of our powers – are hard to imagine, scary, awesome. But equally awesome is the skill of doctors, the compassion of nurses and carers, the empathy of those we love, and the sustaining hope in the Love that will not let us go.

We are human before we are Christian, with all our human vulnerability, and to be Christian is to become more fully human. It is not to lose your humanity, but to enhance it. To know that you (and everyone else) are made in the image of God makes us more human, not less. And it is the all-too-human feelings of anxious apprehension that are met, and more than met, by the assurance that each of us, with our own unique identity, is precious to God. That, in some mysterious way, without us he will be incomplete. Though to be persuaded of that truth will never quite silence those questioning fears when 'the bright day is done,/ And we are for the dark'.[94]

24th September
Use a Shopmobility scooter to negotiate my way through the Salisbury crowds. Rare spurts at 4 m.p.h. A wheelchair is

a healthy lesson in the way we ignore the disabled. A minority notice you and make way: most are unaware of your presence. Though I feel somewhat bogus when I park outside Ottakar's or Waterstone's and move round on two perfectly good legs. It's the energy that's missing. In odd moments, in this waiting state, between recovery from the body's battering in hospital and the threatened unpleasant side-effects of radiation, I'm tempted to self-pity. Then I read this morning of Martine, aged 32, who lost both legs above the knee and was the last person to be brought out from the Aldgate tube bomb having seen horrors that will live with her for life, and it is quickly silenced.

Long-tailed tits pass through the garden most days now, pausing at the dying, bug-infested apple-tree.

25th–26th September: Reflecting on time and eternity ... and prayer (3)

I've written, here and elsewhere, of the significance of our uniqueness – and that of each leaf and snowflake, each single beetle of the 30,000 different species found in one small corner of the Amazon forest. No two words, depending on their context, are ever quite the same, nor will they be heard in absolutely identical ways. No two moments, in which new choices face us, can ever be identical either. Each is unique and unrepeatable. What does this signify for our understanding of time? St Augustine wrote:

> Time can only be coming from the future, passing through the present, and going into the past. In other words, it is coming out of what does not yet exist, passing through what has no duration, and moving into what no longer exists. What, then is time? If no one asks of me, I know; if I wish to explain it to him who asks, I don't know.

When William Blake wrote of doing good in 'minute particulars', I hear him speaking both of the infinite care with which, in any given moment, we must exercise love, but

193

also of the rash and exotic variety of the created world and its swarming existence that cries out to be noticed.

One of the themes of Eliot's *Four Quartets* is how we may triumph over the straitjacket of time and discover 'the still point' at the heart of the dance, the 'unattended moment'. For him history is 'a pattern of timeless moments'. We may try to escape from time by ignoring its implacable passage until it pulls us up sharply with a reminder that the sands in the hour-glass run much more swiftly towards the end.

How may we, even in this life, just occasionally attain a sense of timelessness, experience (as it were) the other side of time? By learning to *be* rather than *do* is easily said. It has to do with renunciation, with self-surrender, the letting-go of worldly possessions and achievements, which should come more easily with old age; but also by understanding that the events which we claim to be central to faith – Incarnation, Passion and Crucifixion – happened within time but *they also transcend it*. They straddle time and eternity. So it has to do with seeing what Eliot calls 'sudden illuminations', those small epiphanies in which you lose yourself and which people in every generation have believed to be a brief and fragmentary awareness of the God who is outside time, and who (in Augustine's words) 'made the world not *in* time but *with* time'. 'All transient things', wrote Thomas Traherne, 'are permanent in God.'

Unlike God, whose 'time' we call 'eternity', we can only exist in time, in this particular moment, and we can only discern God in what Pere de Caussade called 'the sacrament of the present moment ... [Leaving] the past to the infinite mercy of God, the future to his good providence ... [giving] the present wholly to his love by being faithful to his grace.'[95] Most moments in our lives are predictable and humdrum, for otherwise life would be impossible, yet there are some moments that turn out to be momentous. (For the grunion fish, its biological clock dictating the movements of all living things, there is one day in the year when the time is right for spawning, and thousands of them reach the shore of a particular beach in California, not only on the same day each year, but within a period of two hours – what someone had described as 'the date you don't want to miss'.) For us, in a flash, while the world goes about its business, an accident happens; on an otherwise normal day cancer is diagnosed, a child is born, we exchange marriage vows, a loved one dies; and our world is never the same again. But if we have learned how to give attention (the kind of attention we may give to a book, a play or a concert, or when painting or shaping clay, when for a while you are taken out of yourself and time seems to contract), if we know how to observe and to listen, then in every passing moment and every casual encounter we have the potential to be open to whoever or whatever is before us. Then there may be a small shift in our perception of each other, or we may see some new beauty created by a different fall of light. Walter Pater said that 'it is only the roughness of the eye' that makes 'any two persons, things, situations seem alike'.

If we were truly alive to the texture of things, the look and the feel of them, and the fragmentary nature of the world, how long would it take to appreciate a bowl of fruit? The Irish poet, Patrick Kavanagh, wrote of how all civilisations are built on parochialism:

> To know fully even one field or one land is a lifetime's experience. In the world of poetic experience it is depth that counts, not width. A gap in a hedge, a smooth rock surfacing a narrow lane, a view of a woody meadow, the stream at the junction of four small fields – these are as much as a man can fully experience.[96]

And the Scottish poet Don Paterson, in a book of reflections and aphorisms, echoes this when he writes of how in his life the time when he has actually lived 'in the present moment' would amount to no more than a single day:

> If only I could have lived it as a single day; it would have thrown its light onto all the others, like a brazier in a dark

arcade. Instead I find my way by sparks, and what they briefly make visible.[97]

Theologians and philosophers are intrigued by the paradox of time and eternity, and with the difference of what the New Testament calls *kairos* and *chronos*. *Chronos* is something to be measured by the ticking of the clock. In spring and autumn we cheat on clock time by adding or gaining an hour, making time flow backwards. *Kairos* is what we mean by such phrases as 'the time is ripe', indicating a time of opportunity or fulfilment – those significant moments in our lives which demand a decision and bring about change. (As in the words in Ecclesiastes about 'a time to be born, and a time to die; a time to plant and a time to pluck up that which is planted ...') The Old Testament prophets look forward to the time when the Messiah will be revealed, and the birth of Jesus, in the words of U. A. Fanthorpe's poem 'BC/AD':

... was the moment
When a few farm workers and three
members of an obscure Persian sect
Walked haphazard by starlight straight
Into the kingdom of heaven.
This was the moment when Before
Turned into After ...[98]

When he comes for baptism John declares that 'the time is fulfilled'. In those moments of birth and baptism – and all the subsequent moments of healing, affirming, suffering, dying and rising – the eternal breaks into time, the Kingdom is begun, and time is revealed as the imposter we allow it to be when we imagine that our allotted ration of birthdays is all that life amounts to. For beneath every passing moment there lies a moment of a different kind, a reality of a changed quality. It is as if, in acknowledging our relationship in Christ with the One in whom we have always lived and moved and had our being, we are grounding ourselves in a moment that is timeless, not just *chronos* but *kairos* too, one which speaks of eternity. Richard Crashaw writes of the nativity as 'all wonders in one sight/ Eternity shut in a span'.[99] Eliot writes of 'timeless moments'; Meister Eckhart of 'the eternal Now'; Kierkegaard of our need 'to cram today with eternity and not with the next day', and wondering how Jesus lived his final days 'without anxiety', believes it was because 'he had eternity with him in the day that is called today, and therefore the next day had no power over him, it had no existence for him'; and William Blake spoke of holding 'Infinity in the palm of your hand,/ And Eternity in an hour'.

John Taylor, in *The Go-Between God*, presents us with a striking image. Do we see ourselves, set in the living stream of history and the moment that is *now*, as facing the downstream flow, so that our 'now' is coming from behind us and carrying with it all the debris from the past? If so, we are imprisoned in the contradiction between what is and what might have been. Or do we picture ourselves facing upstream, so that our 'now' is always coming to meet us, for then our task is to rise to the challenge of what is and what might be. The first way, however realistic, contains nothing of hope or expectation. If we claim the title of 'the Easter people', then it's the second way that rings true to the promises of Jesus. John Taylor quotes Jürgen Moltmann writing of the Resurrection:

> It is without parallel in the history known to us. But it can for that very reason be regarded as a 'history-making event' in the light of which all other history is illumined, called in question and transformed.[100]

No human being witnessed the Resurrection of Jesus, just the effect it had on those who came to believe in it. Look directly at the sun and you will be blinded, but by its light everything is transformed. For Paul, Jesus is the first-fruits of a new creation, and the Cross and Resurrection enable us to see the future with new hope. That ultimate demonstration of the nature and cost of self-giving love has set us free from the past.

What, then, does it mean to live in Eckhart's 'eternal Now', to live without anxiety? Kierkegaard defined 'anxiety' as 'dread' and likened it to dizziness, the 'dizziness of freedom which occurs when freedom gazes down into its own possibility'. By which he means what the New Testament means when it describes us as being 'strangers and pilgrims on the earth', and what Augustine means by being 'restless until we rest in thee'. The world can be a hostile place. Bad things happen to everyone. Yet it is this very anxiety, this restlessness, which may prompt my search for God. And implicit in that word 'search' is the fact that I am not only self-aware but incomplete, open to possibility, able to choose, to decide from moment to moment how to respond, how to act, what to say; and that each day is infinitesimally (but maybe crucially) different from the one that precedes it.

So here I am, not just a product of my genes and rather strange upbringing,[101] but desiring to become the person God created me to be, believing that (paradoxically) to desire to serve him is Cranmer's 'perfect freedom'. And that includes the freedom to live without anxiety. Trapped by time, daily a little nearer death, yet 'having eternity with me in the day that is called today' because I have faith that I am (in Christ) in a relationship with One whom daily I call 'Abba, Father', One who moment by moment gives life to all that exists. This is to see life with a kind of dual vision: with one pair of eyes fixed on the temporal, the ever-present world where the possibilities are increasingly limited by the ageing body, and with a second pair of eyes to see time as a human invention masking a more profound reality, the eternal hidden presence of God. Sight transfigured by insight. The anxiety of life's unpredictability transformed by trust in the changeless, undergirding Love.

Whenever I use that loveliest of Cranmer's collects which ends with the plea that 'we may so pass through things temporal that finally we lose not the things eternal' (which survives in *Common Worship*: Trinity 4), I remember one of those to whom I've dedicated this book, for he and his wife said it each evening during the final months of his life. Paul writes that our eyes should be fixed 'not on the things that are seen, but on the things that are unseen: for what is seen passes away; what is unseen is eternal'.[102] The 'now' and the 'not yet' of the Kingdom: small signs of it everywhere for those with eyes to see, but its full flowering in some unimaginable future. Most of the time I'm unaware of 'the moment under the moment'. None of us ever could live in the 'eternal Now'. 'The world is too much with us.' And yet ... if you live with someone you love and trust and gradually come to know and love ever more deeply, you're not constantly analysing the relationship. Most of the time you take it for granted, a kind of silent, shared heartbeat.

Yet there are moments when you are aware of how it has changed and enriched your life. Not just bits of it, but all of it. Similarly, to be 'in Christ', to seek to share his trustful openness to the Father, is to know at your deep centre the enduring melody of his love for you. And there are ways of living out this truth. By taking time; by consciously setting aside those unattended moments when we are content to be rather than to do. Becoming aware of everything in your body working in perfect harmony to hold you in being: heart and lungs and nerves and blood and brain all working to sustain you, to repair what is damaged and (speaking personally) to learn how to be a mouth rather than a leg, its cells slowly adapting over the months from thigh cells to mouth cells. To expose ourselves to the magic of words or paint and the hidden power of music. Taking time to notice the shape of trees in winter, the pattern on leaf and bark, the feel of stones, the way clouds form, or how a flock of starlings moves as one. To give attention and listen to the person met by chance in those unlooked for encounters that may only happen once. To take time for that form of prayer (alone or with others) which centres on silence and stillness, and which may grow out of the slow repetition of certain familiar words which we have found speak to us of the things of the spirit.

It may not happen often, but to open ourselves in this way can bring a deeper sense of the God who is to be found (as Gandhi said) 'in the next person you meet or not at all'; permeating his creation, not remote and removed from it; in experiences of desolation as well as in times of delight; and in the moment that is Now and not in some unguessable future heavenly melange of harps and haloes. It's what the playwright Dennis Potter described, in viewing plum blossom frothing beneath the window of the room in which he was dying of cancer: of how things which have seemed important become trivial and what you have hardly noticed becomes important, 'and the difference between the trivial and the important doesn't seem to matter, but the nowness of everything is absolutely wondrous ...'[103] Where such ordinary moments carry with them a sense of the extra-ordinary, they seem to contain a kind of validity which can then carry over into the rest of our lives. John Stewart Collis writes in his *Autobiography*:

> I saw that no 'materialistic' explanation of life could deprive it of its glory, since the material is as immaterial as the material, the ordinary as extraordinary as the extraordinary, the natural as supernatural as the supernatural, while the miracle of water is as great as any turning of water into wine. It occurred to me that the answer to the riddle of the world is to be able to *see* the world; and that instead of worrying about salvation we should recognise that vision *is* salvation.[104]

The common definition of religion is in terms of morality: 'do this', 'don't do that'. Look up the word 'Christian' in the American *Thesaurus of Slang* and you find the following extraordinary synonyms: 'white, respectable, good egg, square toes [?], steady man'. But Christianity is to be understood simply and solely in terms of a *relationship of love* which, once entered into, changes you – and has the power to go on changing you, however frustratingly slowly – as responding to being loved always must. That relationship is the framework in which the rest of my life is set and which determines its values and its direction. That relationship, however, is more than just a personal relationship to a supreme Being, absolute in power and goodness. For, as Bonhoeffer wrote, 'it implies a new life for others, through participation in the being of God ... A life based on the transcendent.'[105] I see prayer as a recognition and a reminder: the recognition of each moment's potential; the reminder that the physical and the spiritual, the visible and the invisible, interpenetrate each other and are part of a single vision. A reminder, too, that there is no moment in which I can't express my need, my penitence, my desire for the welfare and happiness of others, and my gratitude. Above all, my gratitude.

27th September

Reflecting further on Gandhi's words about the God who is to be found 'in the next person you meet', and William Blake's 'he who would do good to another must do it in Minute Particulars', of how we can only tackle the world's problems one thing – one person – at a time, I'm reminded of the story of the American anthropologist, Loren Eiseley, told in a book of essays read years ago and long since gone the way of all paperbacks. He was walking on a beach, full of starfish which had been flung onto the sand by the huge waves. He meets a young man whom he names 'the star thrower'. Where the star thrower finds a living starfish he picks it up and flings it far into the sea. Eiseley points out that the beach goes on for miles. There must be thousands of starfish. He won't be able to save them all before the heat of the morning sun kills them. How can the saving of a few make any difference? The man picks up another starfish and throws it far into the waves. 'To this one,' he says, 'it makes a difference.'

28th–29th September: Reflecting on words (5) ...
and the power of stories

John McGahern in his fine *Memoir* writes of how 'There are
no days more full in childhood than those days that are not
lived at all, the days lost in a book.'[106] Which prompts me to
add a postscript on the hidden power of words – or rather,
stories. For centuries people's experience of the world was
incarnated in stories, and time has done nothing to diminish
their power. If as children we have had a passion for books to
ameliorate our loneliness and give wing to our imagination,
there are certain stories that we remember all our lives. For
me, that meant fairy tales from the Brothers Grimm and the
legendary Aesop; tales of Babar and Winnie the Pooh, Alice
and Long John Silver and Toad. These were followed by the
adventures of William and his gang and Biggles, the shining
heroes of the wartime comics, and the rather tiresome children of Arthur Ransome's *Swallows and Amazons* families, for
whose future Rockfist Rogan of the RAF in my weekly *Hotspur*
was risking his charmed life. Now they've mostly been
superceded by tales of Harry Potter and Philip Pullman's
Lyra, Tolkein's Frodo and Bilbo Baggins and the children of
Narnia. The stories transport their readers to a magical world
that sparks their sense of wonder and engages them in the
age-old battle between good and evil. It's one of the ways in
which we learn to distinguish between them and are helped
to form our own values and priorities.

While some treat the stories that form the framework of
the Bible with a literalism that distorts their purpose, others
dismiss them as no more than fairy-tales from a bygone age.
I wrote on 23rd August about the distinction between *logos*
and *mythos*, and the true meaning of myth. Truth is complex
and may be conveyed in more subtle, less literalist ways
than the scientific. When the writers of Genesis want a story
about the sovereignty of God, our role as stewards of creation and the way we abuse his gift of freedom, a story that
will lodge in the mind and capture the imagination of a
child or a Milton, they use powerful images of a man and a

woman, a talking snake, an apple and a garden. A theological explanation of the gifts and risks attached to free will would have left us cold (as it may do when Paul struggles to explain the difference between law and grace in his Letter to the Galatians), but a story can be unforgettable, a universal myth conveying universal truths. And when Jesus says, 'There was once a man who had two sons' or 'Somebody lost a sheep' or 'This man went down from Jerusalem to Jericho', no one dreams of asking whether it 'really happened'. All that matters is whether the story makes its deeper point and illustrates a general and timeless truth about God and us which can be told or painted in memorable words and images. It is as 'true' as today's newspaper account of the old man ejected for mild heckling yesterday at the Labour Party Conference. This conveying of truth through made-up stories, providing images for the imagination as well as words for the intellect, had been part of the contemporary Graeco-Roman world, and it has always been an effective tool in Judaism. History was written, not so much for information, as to convey a certain viewpoint, a religious or ethical truth.

There is an account in the Book of Acts of a lame man who is cured when he hears from Peter 'the story of Jesus'. Not in this case a made-up story conveying a significant truth, but Peter's account of events he had witnessed which had changed both their lives. Martin Buber writes about the potential a story has, both to convey a new truth and also to bring about such a change and liberate those who hear it. For the lame man was no doubt cured of more than his gammy leg. Martin Buber tells this story:

My grandfather was paralysed. One day he was asked to tell about something that happened with his teacher – the great Baalschem. He told how the saintly Baalschem used to leap about and dance while he was at his prayers. As he went on with the story my grandfather stood up; he was so carried away that he had to show how the master had done it, and started to caper about and dance. From that moment on he was cured. That is how stories should be told.[107]

I'm trying to live one day at a time, in what the Americans call 'the nowness of the now'. It's not easy. Mouth very inflamed, still struggling to come to terms with the refashioned jaw. Buy a new watch, guaranteed 'to last a lifetime': a small challenge to the remaining cancer. Though it's an absurd claim. Lifetimes, like pieces of string, are of unpredictable lengths.

30th September

Will the Royal Mail survive in the age of e-mails and rapid technological change? Over 400 cards and letters since mid-July have been a lifeline: tangible proof of affection, prayer and concern, that can't be erased at the touch of a 'delete' key. Letter from Fred B. this morning. He writes, 'I remember you almost every day.' I warm to the honesty of that 'almost'.

2nd October: Reflecting on the meaning of mercy

To Roche Court, the nearby sculpture garden/art gallery, to revisit Antony Gormley's standing steel figures, now turned a rich rust by the rain and dew, Richard Long's *Buzzard*, its flight-path to a distant tree a line of Norfolk flints, and Barbara Hepworth's polished marble figures which always seem to be lit from within; all of them with much else placed with skill in the large, handsome garden with its long view over the Wiltshire countryside. Open daily, free. We go there often. It's what a gallery should be, a refreshment for the spirit.

This morning's set Psalm (136) is the only one which in the second half of every verse repeats the words unchanged: 'and his mercy endures for ever'. 'Mercy', a word that occurs a hundred times in the Psalms and fifty times elsewhere in the Old Testament. When Coverdale translated the Hebrew word *hesed* he sometimes used 'mercy' and sometimes 'lovingkindness' to communicate God's tender compassion for his creatures. In his *City of God* Augustine defined mercy as 'heartfelt sympathy for another's distress, impelling us to succour him if we can', and Thomas Aquinas wrote that 'mercy takes its name "misericordia" (*miserum cor*) from a person's compassionate heart for another's unhappiness'. The first revelation of what became the Koran (or Qur'an), sacred to the one in five human beings who are Muslim, was given to the sixth-century prophet Muhammad when he was meditating in a mountain cave outside Mecca. Fearful of the experience, he was taken by his wife to a Christian cousin, who assured him – when he recited the beginning of what he had heard – that it was of the same Truth as that brought by Moses and Jesus. Muhammad and his followers were persecuted for their seeming heresy. After an attempt was made on his life, he and his fellow-Muslims fled from Mecca in 622, which became known as the Year of the Emirates, the year from which all years in Islamic history are counted.

'Whithersoever ye turn', claims the Koran, 'there is the Face of God.' Like the Bible, the Koran has been – and is being – used indiscriminately and piecemeal by certain Islamic fundamentalists, in this case to justify violence against non-Muslims as part of the 'holy war', the *jihad*. Yet each part of the Koran begins with the words that reflect the spirit of the whole: 'In the name of God, the compassionate, the merciful.' Compassion and mercy: two words which are the starting-point for all our thinking about the nature of God and against which all other claims to truth and insight must be tested. Words which unite the three great Abrahamic faiths of Judaism, Christianity and Islam. Perhaps 'the enduring melody' is at root 'the enduring mercy'.

Watch ITV's *Elizabeth I* with Helen Mirren as the Queen. It includes the beheading of Mary, Queen of Scots. Strange to think of how I worshipped daily within a stone's throw of both their tombs erected by James I, one each side of the Abbey's Lady Chapel. The TV version omits the most poignant detail of Mary's execution: the story of how her pet dog was afterwards found hidden in her skirts. Robert Wynkfield, who was present, vouches for it: after the execution 'it would not depart from the dead corpse, but came and lay between her head and her shoulders'. Of dogs, Martin Luther wrote (rather surprisingly): 'Be comforted, little dog; thou too at the resurrection shall have a little golden tail.'

4th October

An infected tooth isn't helping the tender state of my mouth. To the dentist for deep root canal treatment, part one. Ronnie Barker, most gifted of actor/comedians is dead. Glad that we met him a couple of years ago and were able to thank him for so much delight over some 40 years. A good tribute from Ronnie Corbett. The latter and I were (non-flying) fellow pilot officers at RAF Hornchurch in 1950, and I found recently an indignant note he sent me when my puppy ate a pair of his leather gloves. It died not long afterwards. Listen to Mahler's great *Resurrection Symphony*. Brings back memories of an evening at the P.'s mountain house in the hills of North Carolina, remote enough to sit outside on the balcony and watch the sun set over Table Rock while Mahler's music exploded all around us.

5th October: Reflecting on mystery

How unaware I am of the subtle, unimaginably complex, mystery of the minute-by-minute functioning of my body as I pick up my pen and begin to write. My immune system may be diminished, yet everything is working to repair and restore what is damaged and reconstructed by the surgeons. The radiotherapy will be invasive, destroying good as well as infected tissue, but the body's inbuilt capacity to heal itself remains. Some scientists give the impression that within a generation we shall know all that we need to know about the physical universe. Even dark matter? The latest research reveals some wonderfully paradoxical facts. It acts as a kind of cosmic glue, holding the galaxies together, and is thought to make up 23 per cent of the universe, compared with 4 per cent of 'normal' matter that can be seen and felt. According to Cambridge's Institute of Astronomy, dark matter has a temperature exceeding that on the suface of the sun, yet it does not give off any heat. Particles of it zip about at 9 km per second, are loosely packed, transparent and have no electric charge, yet are weighty enough to exert a gravitational pull that prevents the stars and galaxies from flying apart.

Nor is it only the mystery of the galaxies that still defeats us, but the behaviour of the tiniest particles, and the brain that observes them both. Carl Sagan, Professor of Astronomy and Space Sciences at Cornell University, claims that an all-embracing knowledge 'within a generation' is not only unlikely but, given the capacity of the human brain, impossible. He asks whether we can know, 'ultimately and every detail', a grain of salt. One microgram of table salt, a single just visible speck, contains 10^{16} atoms of sodium and chlorine. That's a 1 followed by 16 zeros, 10 million billion atoms. To say nothing of the forces holding these atoms together. And each atom, rank upon rank of them, are 'in an ordered array, a regularly alternating structure – sodium, chlorine, sodium, chlorine ...' In the brain there are perhaps 10^{11} neurons: that's to say, the circuit elements and switches responsible through their electrical and chemical activity for the way our minds function. Just one brain neuron has some thousand little wires (dendrites) which connect it with its fellow-neurons. It's thought that every bit of information that we take into our brains corresponds to one of these connections. So, concludes Sagan, the total number of things knowable by the brain is no more than 10^{14}, 100 thousand billion. That's just 1 per cent of the number of atoms in that grain of salt, which helps put our hope of understanding our universe into perspective. And, of course, no two grains of salt, any more than two fingerprints, are exactly alike.

I don't find the grains of salt argument wholly persuasive.

The much more powerful human analogy is that, while scientists understand more and more about the how and why of human life and behaviour, yet it is still only a small part; and those tiny differences in our DNA make it impossible for a human brain to know intimately all the people in the world or any one of them completely. Science is the search for rules, and much about our universe is knowable, but not entirely so. And it's just because the natural laws governing our universe are not totally regular or predictable; because human consciousness is deeply mysterious and the human spirit defies definition; because we live in a universe of quantum mechanics, dark matter and black holes; because light seems to consist (inexplicably) sometimes of waves, sometimes of particles; and because to have a sense of the transcendent, as Wittgenstein observed, is to know that 'the facts of the world are not the end of the matter'; that I believe we shall always have to settle for Paul's seeing 'through a glass darkly' or Isaac Newton's sense, at the end of his life, of having been

> ... a boy playing on the sea-shore, and diverting myself in now and then finding a smoother pebble or a prettier shell than ordinary, while the great ocean of truth lay all undiscovered before me.[108]

Carl Sagan welcomes a universe in which much is knowable and much unknown and, indeed, unknowable:

> A universe in which everything is known would be static and dull, as boring as the heaven of some weak-minded theologians. A universe that is unknowable is no fit place for a thinking being. The ideal universe for us is one very much like the universe we inhabit. And I would guess that this is not really much of a coincidence.[109]

7th October

I recognise that this cancer journey has (all too humanly) increased my desire to pray. But will it last? I love Hosea's words in which he speaks of God's justice, which 'dawns like the morning star, its dawning as sure as the sunrise' and which will 'come down to us like the showers, like the spring rains that water the earth', and compares it with our love for God, which is 'like the morning mist, like the dew that goes early away'.[110] And God's desire? Trust. And loyalty.

8th October

Letter from the 84-year-old Ronald Blythe in Wormingford. The best letter-writer I know. Says he spends much time 'just watching, which is what writers do. [The novelist] William Sansom gave "watching" as his hobby in *Who's Who*.' The result? Books like *Akenfield*, articles and private letters, which are full of acute perception, a deep love of nature, and non-judgemental affection for people which together add up to wisdom. R. also writes:

> I have tried to imagine what (your illness) could have been like, for there is no greater chasm than that which exists between the sick and the – so far as they know – healthy. Imagination cannot bridge it, though love might now and then take a flying leap towards such suffering.

The operative word is 'tried'.

9th October

Mouth very sore and radiotherapy starting this week. Makes me feel pretty sorry for myself. Self-pity is an unattractive, negative emotion, and is at once silenced by reading today of the desperate state of Pakistan following the massive earthquake. Self-pity is quite different from self-love, that proper regard for your own value, without which (Jesus implied) the love of neighbour won't happen. If only we could realise that it's a kind of blasphemy to view ourselves with so little compassion when God views us with so much, a form of doubting the divine judgement.

And not just Pakistan silences my complaining. Garri Holness, the last survivor pulled out of the most seriously wrecked underground carriage in the London bombings, who lost part of his leg, says that he now wants each day of the rest of his life 'to be beautiful'. Some challenge! Human beings ache for beauty, though we find it hard to define. There is the beauty of musical harmony, of architectural proportion, of the natural world, of the human body; the beauty of character and of certain faces. Glimpses of beauty and grace may be heartbreaking and momentarily move us to tears. Or even to jealousy, as in Iago's rage that Othello 'has a daily beauty in his life/ That makes me ugly'. Garri Holness's desire no doubt relates to beauty as the absolute contrast to his searing experience in that wrecked train, surrounded by broken, mutilated human beings. Beauty hints at a kind of perfection and order that we search for all our lives, that yearning for harmony and wholeness of which it is an intimation. In recognising beauty we are recognising and affirming how we should like life to be and how we should like to be too. It's a kind of presentiment of heaven. 'Beauty,' wrote Stendhal, 'is the promise of happiness.' And its source? Augustine answers that:

> Ask the beauty of the earth, the beauty of the sea, the beauty of the sky. Question the order of the stars, the sun whose brightness lights the day, the moon whose splendour softens the gloom of night. Ask of the living creatures that move in the waves, that roam the earth, that fly in the heavens. Question all these and they will answer, 'Yes, we are beautiful.' Their very loveliness is their confession of God: for who made these lovely mutable things, but he who is himself unchangeable beauty?[111]

The diarist Francis Kilvert, who was to die in his thirties, was once asked why he had kept his incomparable diary of events and people and the changing face of nature. He replied,

> Partly because life seems to me such a curious and wonderful thing that it almost seems a pity that a humble and uneventful

210

life as mine should pass altogether away without some such
record as this ... It is such a luxury to be alive.

So much for self-pity.

10th October
To Southampton. My mask is tested and marked up for the
radiotherapy. Told to keep absolutely still, eyes forced shut,
plastic ball wedged in my mouth. Lights flash on and off,
lasers play on me, machines whirr, a pen scratches my mask
and lips. Lie still for 45 minutes: it seems an eternity. At first
I grunt at the repeated words, 'All right?' but soon realise
they're not addressed to me. No indication of how long it
will take and no word to me throughout. I want to mutter,
'There's a human being in here.' First and single (and
therefore all the more noticeable) instance of the lack of
what lies at the heart of good treatment: communication.
Southampton has this wonderful new radiotherapy/oncol-
ogy centre costing millions of pounds, yet the hospital,
seriously in the red, is forbidden to spend money on replacing staff. Those arriving via the main hospital (as almost all
do at the first visit) wend their way through the corridors but
find no receptionist in the waiting room to greet patients:
you wait to be called. In a cancer centre, where many arrive
anxious, a welcoming face is reassuring. (*Later:* following
A.'s letter, they write to say that this is to be put right 'very
shortly'.) And how odd that, in a place of healing, the first
shop you see is a Burger King.

11th October
At the eleventh hour, an hour of deep root canal at dentist's.
After the operation, what might have seemed daunting, no
longer does.

12th October
In Kashmir, following the earthquake, in what was Bagh's
sixth-form college for more than 1500 students, people were

211

heard calling for help. For four days the trapped teenagers cried out, but rescuers only had their bare hands with which to dig and gradually the cries ceased. All are now dead. As a makeshift memorial the villagers placed alongside the ruins exercise books and diaries found in the rubble. One had fallen open at the words: 'Language: the way we express our thoughts.' But no words could have expressed the thoughts of those students as they slowly awaited their deaths.

To Southampton for the first radiotherapy session. Another 40-minute session strapped to the table in the tight-fitting mask, whilst they plot the computer with the exact path the radiation will take over the next seven weeks.

13th October
The daily trip to hospital starts in earnest. We opt for the route via Romsey, almost wholly on country roads. It's a late autumn, many trees only just beginning to turn. Loveliest are the single silver maples, their leaves varying from green to deep lemon and russet. No frosts yet to scatter their leaves. By the time of our last trip no doubt all the leaves will have fallen.

14th October
A. sees a learner in town in a driving-school car. Sticker in back window says: 'Put Jesus in the driving-seat.' Driver doing a very hesitant 20 m.p.h.

15th–16th October
Our Ruby Wedding weekend. Had planned to be at South-wark Cathedral (where we got married) for the Sunday Eucharist, but we were over-optimistic. On Saturday to the family in Earley for a wonderful lunch party: family and close friends, 22 of us. Find it extraordinary to think that, if I hadn't married Alison, five of them – and more in the future – simply wouldn't exist. Procreating really is the most significant thing we ever do, and we should be amazed by it if it weren't so common. A day for deep gratitude.

17th October

J., radiographer, observing the hairs in my mouth from my transplanted leg, says the radiation will deal with them. Tells me of a patient who had skin taken from his upper arm and who now has half a naked woman on his palate.

19th October

Spectacular day. Driving to Southampton the sun shone on the bronze, green, pale orange and gold of the autumnal trees against a Wagnerian background of a bruised, gunmetal sky. Heavy showers, flooded roads. Driving home, great mountainous heaps of shining cumulus, lit from behind. In the far distance the thin cathedral spire. Noticeably less energy, increasingly sore mouth. Two hours at clinic, one of the three machines having broken down. I lie trapped in the unyielding plastic for 15 minutes a day – though they have now cut holes for my eyes. Meditate on the paradox of the radiation healing by destroying, both the bad tissue and the healthy.

21st October

A combination of cumulus and cirrus clouds, the sky looking as if a child has been let loose with a packet of grey and white crayons. Good piece in the *Guardian* by the humanist Bernard Crick applauding some recent lectures by Rowan Williams, and pleading for humanists to be less fussy about working with the religious as both share a common commitment to justice. Cites an inter-faith body in East London, the Citizens' Organising Foundation, made up of Christians of many traditions, Jews, Muslims and Hindus, who campaign on issues of poverty, discrimination and empowerment, whose actions are energized by a morality of social justice. He was proud (as a former Vice-President of the British Humanist Association) to be made an honorary fellow at a service at St Martin-in-the-Fields. Differing motivations but common action.

Three months since my operation. Body check: mouth

sore, tongue ulcerated, 'flap' still very swollen, as are the chin and neck; left ear, shoulder and thigh feel bruised and partially numb; energy level lower again; spirits reasonably high, dipping by early evening; taste returning. Could be so much worse.

23rd October

As chairman of the local support group for the Medical Foundation for the Care of Victims of Torture, I had invited Patricia Routledge to present a one-woman evening at Salisbury Playhouse. I was to interview her about her life for 45 minutes, and then she would perform. In the event I just have enough energy (and voice) to welcome and introduce her to a packed house, warm and sympathetic from the start. She is by chance on a set for Ayckbourn's *Woman in Mind*, a suburban garden which, with its genteel border of polyanthus and dinky fence, is not unlike Hyacinth Bucket's. She ranges from Alan Bennett's first *Talking Heads* monologue (which he wrote for her) to a moving Mistress Quickly on the death of Falstaff, heard in rapt stillness. She sups with us afterwards. Makes my day by picking up one of my more successful pottery side-plates and enquiring, 'Bernard Leach?'

25th October

Ten of the thirty-two radiotherapy sessions under my belt. See duty doctor as mouth already extremely ulcerated, and it's hard even to eat the blandest puréed food. It has never really recovered from all the toxins my body has taken in during the past months. The tablets ranged in the bathroom grow daily. Stop on the main road to Romsey to let a herd of Friesian cows cross in their vague, stop-go way.

27th October

A glorious, warm, cloudless, autumnal day, the countryside transformed. Mouth feels as if it is one gigantic ulcer. On painkillers day and night and 20 sessions still to come. Begin to understand C.B.'s remark that the radiation process will be 'as demanding as the operation'. Gandhi, my South Indian radiologist, says severe burning and ulceration is normal with radiation of the mouth. J. the radiation nurse, about to go on holiday for a fortnight in the sun: 'See you two weeks on Monday – by which time you'll be feeling *really* horrible!' Thank you, J. Among the things I neither want nor need to know, that rates pretty high.

28th October
Can't conceive what 'really horrible' will be like if this isn't it. Can't talk, barely able to eat. Write endless notes to A. What do I pray for? 'Endurance', I guess. And the avoidance of tiresome self-pity.

29th October
Shan't be writing much for a while. Weekends free from radiotherapy should be a relief, but even the daily trip to Southampton gives a shape to the day, and each dose is a day nearer the end. Just read that the average age of death for men is 76.2 years. I make that Wednesday week.

31st October
C.B. away, so see Registrar at hospital about state of mouth. Even she seems impressed. Put on morphine sooner than they or I would have wished. Food an increasing problem: mashed banana, avocado, yoghurt still just OK, plus porridge, mild soup. Appetite small, which helps, but they're keen I don't lose weight. At a very low point tonight.

2nd November
All Saints' Day and All Souls' Day barely observed. Remembering my parents on the latter is strange. It's complex to pray for a father you can't remember, and when I pray for my mother I wonder how she stands with her three husbands. 'In heaven they neither marry nor are given in marriage', I know, but that can't just turn you into strangers.

Though in her confused old age it was her dogs she remembered rather than her husbands. Halfway stage for radiotherapy. See C.B. back from holiday. Puts me on cocaine mouthwash before meals (*sic*) and ups the morphine. Feel a bit more in control of pain. As we leave, there's a boy of about ten in a wheelchair, quite bald, his head in a holding-frame. Feel ashamed at my complaining. Must add him to my prayers.

3rd November
Only one machine out of three working today. Again a two-hour wait. Collect cocaine mouthwash, issued strictly one week at a time. At meal-time, it numbs the mouth for about four minutes, so eat fast. On the car journey we listen to the CD of *Master and Commander*, turning down the sound during the bloodier descriptions of naval battles and operations on the unaesthetised wounded.

4th November
Trip to Southampton becoming part of our lives. Know every vista, almost every tree, from the posh-sounding Paulette Laclave Avenue to the more homely Bunny Lane, past Broadlands in its grand park and Florence Nightingale's home in Wellow, past the fruit farm, the business park, the garden centre, and Pepperbox Hill. Past the hawk regularly sitting in the highest branch of an oaktree outside Romsey, old-man's-beard crawling along the hedges, the slim poplars the first to shed all their leaves.

7th November
Slow walk by Avon. Two little grebes getting furious with their chick. Long-tailed tits, never staying long. Caroline Waldman drives me today. Too sore to talk in car, so she chooses music she thinks I'll like. Rather riskier than recommending novels. Lovely soft light, but the winds of the past two days have stripped the leaves, with many yet still to turn. Reading D. H. Lawrence's *Letters*. He writes of

the deserted English sea-coast in winter, of a 'flat unfinished world'. with 'a few gulls swinging like a half-born thought'. And of 'a blackbird singing' (in the dawn light) 'as if his singing were a sort of talking to himself, or of thinking aloud his strongest thoughts'.

9th November
Two definitions:

> 1. *Mouth:* n. external orifice in head, with cavity behind it containing apparatus of biting and mastication and vocal organs; this cavity.
>
> 2. *Mouth:* n. external orifice in head, much restored: top half, original, bottom half formerly thigh, containing a very few top teeth, useless for biting or masticating; severely ulcerated, surviving saliva glands struggling to produce thick, salty-tasting mucus night and day.

Vocal chords undamaged, but reluctant to speak. Cleaning of teeth out of the question. A dozen sessions to go. No longer need to shave ever again except partly on right-hand side of face. But if it is killing the cancer it will all be worth it.

At clinic reading diaries and letters, easily interrupted, not just Lawrence but that eccentric cleric Sydney Smith, and William Allingham, friend and confidant of Tennyson.

11th November
A., back from Waitrose, impressed that at 11 a.m. all those serving at the tills got to their feet, the rest of the staff lined up against the wall, and all customers stood in silence to observe the two minutes' remembrance. Doubt if that would have happened in pre-Iraq War times. These are increasingly troublesome days (and nights). Understand now why they warn you that the effects of the radiation are cumulative. The effect of the daily burning, unlike ageing, doesn't happen so slowly as to be unnoticeable, but in a series of sudden steps.

12th November

A golden autumn day. We walk a little at Lake. In the late afternoon sun each blade of grass seems clearly defined and there are deep shadows. One huge field is strung from side to side, and as far as the eye can see, with gleaming strands of spiders' webs, as if wrapped in the finest silk. Have finally lost my taste. Only two weeks to go.

13th November

3 a.m.: 'I can't go on.' 8 a.m.: 'I'll go on.' Later I realise that these are an unconscious echo of the final words of Samuel Beckett's *The Unnameable* in the character's struggle between despair and hope. Epistle set for this Sunday, which I read from bed looking out at the distant spire of the cathedral where A. and so many friends are gathered for the Eucharist, is 1 Thessalonians 5:1–11. The last two verses read:

> [Christ] died for us so that awake or asleep we might live in company with him. Therefore encourage one another, build one another up – as indeed you do.

As indeed they do.

15th November

First Christmas card. A few roses still in bloom in the garden. Morning Psalm: 116:6b–12:

> I was brought very low and [the Lord] helped me.
> Turn again to your rest, O my soul,
>   for the Lord has treated you well.
> For you have rescued my life from death,
>   my eyes from tears and my feet from stumbling ...
> I believed, even when I said, 'I have been brought very low.'
> In my distress I said, 'No one can be trusted'.
> How shall I repay the Lord for all the good things
>   he has done for me?

'No one can be trusted.' Realise that throughout I have put my entire trust in the doctors, consultants and surgeons.

Haven't questioned their judgement – simply been grateful for their expertise. Who else do we trust in this fashion? Very few. Loved ones. Friends, whose loyalty has been proved over long years. Airline pilots. Train drivers. God? Yes, insofar as trust is synonymous with faith. One of those educated guesses on which you bet your life, and which is tested in times of trial. 'Set your troubled hearts at rest,' says Jesus at the end. 'Trust in God always; trust also in me.' 'O Lord, in thee have we trusted', we say in the *Te Deum*; but, being human, we cross our fingers and add, 'let me never be confounded.'

Finish David Lodge's fine and sympathetic novel *Author! Author!* about the (to me) unreadable novelist Henry James.

16th November
Skin scarlet, burned and peeling, inside of mouth (to use my consultant's unprofessional word) 'horrible'. Seven more sessions to go. I score them through daily in black ink, like I used to do at school for the longed-for end of term. Have become very fond of my regular radiographers who do their wretched work with much sympathy and care. Each night brings morphine-induced sleep.

20th November
Neck very inflamed: skin at once painful and a constant irritant. Dreading the further burning the last four days will bring. Can only grunt: once for 'yes', twice for 'no'. Beg the consultant (in writing) to be let off, but the answer is an adamant 'no'. Today is the most perfect late autumn day, heavy frost and mist lifting to reveal a cloudless sky. Drive to the Avon near Trafalgar House. Astonishing colours, late and unexpected, in trees bordering the water: russet and gold and lemon, and the deep crimson of the bare willow stems, all mirrored in the still surface of the wide river.

21st November

See C.B. Thinks I may have hit 'the lowest point'. Explains that a mouth tumour, treated solely by surgery, will more often than not return. So the radiotherapy ('which may or may not have been necessary') is a severe case of belt and braces, an additional disincentive destroying many healthy cells in order to eradicate those tempted to divide. It's a pretty barbarous technique when applied to the most sensitive parts of the body, and no doubt in a few years' time may have been superseded.

24th November

This week we've listened in the car to Simon Armitage's dramatisation of *The Odyssey*. Today Odysseus reaches Ithaca, his beloved homeland, after the 20-year journey from Troy, many of them spent in the arms of Calypso. And today I reach a kind of Ithaca, the longed-for goal after six-and-a-half weeks of radiotherapy. Though it's hard to feel celebratory now that the pain and discomfort of the burning are at their most acute, and may (they warn me now) take a month or so gradually to subside. It isn't the end of the journey by any means, but a very significant landmark.

25th–30th November

A week in which I've discovered that for some the worst is reserved for what is hopefully the final phase. No sense yet of liberation. The radiation has been working away, and all this week life has been nasty, painful and depressing. Even the potent-sounding combination of morphine and cocaine mouthwash proves ineffective in relieving a mouth burned scarlet and a scarred and blistered neck. Food has become something to dread. At night I learn what it means when the Psalmist speaks of 'my tongue cleaves to the roof of my mouth', for little saliva is being produced and I wake hourly and have to gently ease the tongue away from its lethal grip on my palate with warm water. Many short 'arrow' prayers,

220

but the daily office goes unsaid. In prayer, as in everything else, I am once again in the hands of others.

On 28th I.D. fitted me into his impossible schedule and gave me his time and full attention; and again on 30th. Gives me a nebuliser to help the dryness at night.

2nd December

Crazy dream. I telephoned heaven to ask why I seemed to be stuck. What about all these people praying for me?

'You don't seem to understand,' said an anonymous voice, patiently. 'God doesn't just *absorb* all the millions of prayers thrown at him daily. The wonderful thing is that he can listen to everyone at once, but he can only deal with the prayers *one at a time*. They have to be processed.'

'Then everyone has a kind of queue of prayers being processed one-by-one?'

'Yes.'

'Where has he got to in my case?'

'There are 2,130,000 to go.'

Felt reassured that each one counted, though surprised at what seemed like a certain divine tardiness about it all.

Weekly letter from Hugh, always full of interest. Pastor, garden designer, artist, poet, botanist: an enviable supply of gifts, well used. He speaks of 'the Numinous Other with utter goodwill towards us, who gradually marinates our hearts in grace regardless of what sort of nonsense we are making of the externals of our lives'. 'He marinates our hearts in grace.' Lovely phrase: lovely friend.

8th December

A fortnight since the radiotherapy ended. A tough time. There followed a sudden and total loss of energy, leaving me almost as weak as after the operation. Of the small number of saliva glands over half have been removed or zapped, and the remaining ones are struggling. Neck healing slowly with the help of surprisingly effective sunflower cream. Eating still very hard. Today I manage without cocaine mouthwash, which is apparently very addictive. Keep forgetting just how battered and invaded my ancient body has been.

11th December
Still unable to get to cathedral Sunday Eucharist. Today's Epistle, from 1 Thessalonians 5: 'Always be joyful; pray continually; give thanks whatever happens.' How often and how glibly have I read those words to others. Now I must learn afresh to live them.

13th December
No doubt the radiation paralyses the facial nerves and a few weeks later they start to come to life again. Now have quite severe, though intermittent, pain in the right-hand side of the jaw, increasing as the day wears on. Reluctantly back on morphine. Tiresome. Tonight there is a bright ring of narrow cloud at some distance from the moon, covering about a third of the night sky. It forms a perfect circle, the nearly-full moon at its exact centre. Never seen anything like it. Quite different from the usual 'ring round the moon' effect. Wonder if it's a result of the massive black cloud released yesterday after the fire at the Hemel Hempstead oil storage depot. Red letter day: can (very gently) clean my teeth again.

14th December
David Attenborough's series, *The World of Insects*, is as extraordinary as anything he has done. Full of wonder. Tonight it's the world of ants. Am reminded of the story of Mrs Patrick Campbell, leading stage actress at the turn of the last century. An elderly scientist was enthusing about ants: 'They are wonderful little creatures; they have their own police force and their own army.' Terribly bored, she leaned forward with an expression of the utmost interest and said: 'No navy, I suppose?'

17th December: Reflecting on justice (and mercy)
Mark gives me Jonathan Sacks's new book, whereas Sarah arives with the equally welcome latest copy of *Hello*. The Chief Rabbi's work prompts a final postscript on the nature of God's justice and mercy – the form love takes when it is expressed in corporate, social terms. Today the paper has a leader on the meaning of giving to charity and stating that for Christians charity-giving is a duty, 'tied up with their salvation, whether by storing up good works or following the example of Christ'. But that's to start in the wrong place and simply adds to the general impression that heaven is somehow earned by doing good on earth – seen, at its most extreme, in the medieval practice of selling 'indulgences'. For there are two words that cancel each other out: 'earn' and 'love'.

Why does Judaism place such an emphasis on social responsibility, what Jonathan Sacks defines as 'the kindness of (and towards) strangers' which is to be the practice of all true believers? Because what the Jewish law knows as *darkhei shalom*, 'the way of peace', is the universalising of *hesedh*, the Hebrew word which is pivotal to their Scriptures. In seeking to define God, the great world religions all take *hesedh* as their starting-point, the basis for all religious life and practice. For *hesedh* means 'kindness' or, more powerfully, 'love'; love not in the sense of an emotion, but expressed as deed. It's what theologians call 'covenant love', the absolute bond by which (as in marriage) two parties pledge themselves to one another, in what Sacks calls 'an open-ended relationship into an unknown future ... It humanises the world'.[112] It stems from God's covenant with Abraham, with Jacob (who is given the new name, Israel), with Moses the Law-giver and the deliverance from Pharoah, and with Jesus, the new Moses, who makes 'a new covenant', an absolute law of love, with all who choose the way of *hesedh*. In terms of how we relate to God, *hesedh* implies loyalty and trust; it's a love that deepens and grows stronger over time. In terms of relating to each other, it means seeking justice and caring for the sick, the hungry, the refugee, the prisoner and the isolated; it entails care and hospitality. It is this *hesedh*, this freely offered grace and mercy and lovingkindness, that the prophets saw to be the wellspring and motivation of God's very being, and for us it is brought to a fine point – as a magnifying-glass will focus the rays of the sun – in the life and teaching of Jesus. And it is wonderfully spelled-out in Paul's description in 1 Corinthians 13 of that quality of *agape*, which is to lie at the heart of the Christian life.

Christians alone speak of God as Trinity, the doctrine of the altruistic love of God. The nearest we can get to pinning down our experience of God is in terms of a relationship: the One who loves ('the love of the Father'), the One who receives and returns that love and reveals it to us ('the grace of the Son'), and the love between them ('the fellowship of the Holy Spirit'), the belief that the ultimate demand on our lives comes from the one Lord who is sustained by, and who expresses his nature, within the give-and-take of love. For this give-and-take, the Augustinian priest-poet, Padraig J. Daly, uses the lovely image of the power the ocean has gradually to shape the land, its returning tides steady as unconditional love:

> The sea by itself is water merely:
> Its miracle is in its beating against the shore,
> Spreading out across flat sands,
>
> Shifting shingle and stone,
> Flowing over piers and jetties,
> Halting before rock
>
> And falling backward on itself to try again,
> Leaping high in the storm,
> Quietly attacking the very base of land.
>
> And God and God and God are love merely
> Until they find foolish us
> To take love's overflow.[113]

If an authentic Christian (or Jewish or Muslim) life is one lived in response to the *hesedh* of God, a recognition that we love because God first loved us in 'love's overflow', then charitable giving has nothing to do with 'storing up good works' or merely 'following the example of Christ' because we are commanded to do so. For it's the only possible expression of our free response. To claim to be in a relationship of love with the very Source of love and not to share what we enjoy is a nonsense, the ultimate selfishness. And in this context 'earning' a reward makes as much sense as would talk of A. 'earning' my love by cooking my meals, or I hers by having worked to 'earn' a living. The same principle applies in thinking about judgement in terms of a court of law and the evidence of a good life reckoned in terms of balancing good deeds against bad ones. For such a legal context and the compiling of lists makes a mockery of the give-and-take of love, of that *agape* which (in Paul's words) 'keeps no score of wrongs' and which, like faith and hope, 'lasts for ever'. Insofar as we open ourselves to one another (and, in the case of believers, to God) in love and friendship and the recognition of human need, we grow; insofar as we treat the world with carelessness and act as if it centres on us, we are diminished. The unanswered, unanswerable question is whether in the end the *hesedh* of God (who knows how and why some are so damaged and never stand a chance) will win even the most blind among us to himself, or whether he will allow us the ultimate freedom of choosing death rather than life and, like a candle flame starved of oxygen, simply flicker out.

19th December
In a survey of ten-year-olds asking them what was 'the best thing in the world', 'making money and getting rich' came top. 'God' comes in (just) at number 10, though Jesus does better, being just pipped at the post for 'most famous person' by Wayne Rooney.

20th December

To Southampton. See I.D. and C.B., the two consultants whom it would be hard to fault for their care and helpfulness. They think I probably 'touched rock bottom' about a week ago. At the very start I.D. promised me (at my prompting) 'a whisky on Christmas Day'. He thinks he may have been somewhat rash. Mouth improved but still very sensitive. Maybe new teeth by the summer? A diet of soft food palls after so many months. My only complaints at present are the sluggish saliva which makes everything taste salty and metallic (though, praise be, some taste has returned), and a new and total numbness of half my lip and chin which is likely to be permanent.

22nd December

First evening outing for six months. To the cathedral for the candlelit carol service. Nearly 2000 people present last night and again tonight, a few having to be turned away because of health and safety requirements, perhaps a bit too strictly observed. Double choir (boys and girls) singing alternate verses from either end of cathedral for first carols. Very effective. Is there a worse image for heaven than Mrs Alexander's 'Where like stars his children crowned,/ All in white shall stand around'? It's the waiting around that sounds so tedious, like the out-patients' clinic. Unlike the incomparable simplicity of Christina Rossetti's 'In the bleak midwinter' with its marvellous last verse – choir and clergy kneeling round the crib to sing: 'What can I give him, poor as I am? ... What I can I give him./ Give my heart.'

Christmas Day

Drive to the family in Berkshire. Mouth improved enough to make my Communion again. Eat puréed turkey and mashed-up trimmings. To defend I.D.'s honour I drink a *very* watered-down small whisky. Our grandson, 15-year-old Adam, has taken the initiative to launch among a few school friends a 'No presents: no poverty' campaign, has written to

226

all the family asking that instead of presents he should be given money with the aim of paying for a mango plantation in the Third World through OXFAM, costing £1600. He stands firm, receives no gifts, gets interviews in the local paper and on local radio, and by the evening of Christmas Day has made £1100. (*Later:* After a new year concert in his Dad's church on 8th January, they now have a total of £3200, enough to buy two mango plantations.) Can't imagine a teenager taking that sort of action even a few years ago. Very proud of him.

New Year's Eve
So that was 2005. The usual mix of darkness and light: the year of devastation from the tsunami, the Pakistan earthquake, the London bombings, the New Orleans floods, the continuing slaughter in Iraq; balanced by a great outpouring of compassion for their victims, the decommissioning by the IRA, gay and lesbian couples achieving the right to civil partnerships, elections in Iraq, the beginning of debt relief for the poorest nations and of measures to counteract climate change, and for England the winning of a remarkable Test series. For us personally, it also proved a bewildering roller-coaster of a year: knocked flat by the eruption of cancer, upheld by superb professional skill and care and consoled by innumerable acts of kindness. More good things than bad.

Not that any line can be drawn yet. For the past week I'm back (unwillingly) on painkillers, with acute, spasmodic, daily pain in one side of the transplanted bit of the new jaw. They're pretty sure that the pain is neuropathic. Not writing much at present as I'm slowly transcribing all these tens of thousands of words from long-hand onto my computer, hoping it makes sense, resisting the temptation to rewite what at the time it felt like and what seemed proper to share.

Felt grumpy when woken just after midnight by excessively noisy fireworks. A somewhat Scrooge-like way for me to welcome in the new year.

4th January

Imagined I would end this journal with the arrival of 2006, but these are unexpectedly difficult days, and I don't want to end on a down-note. The pain has increased, pinpointed on one side of the 'flap'. Back on morphine four times a day. All part, I'm assured, of the nerves and cells 'settling down'. Feels more like in-fighting.

6th January

Contact clinic as pain still bad. Senior registrar confirms no infection. Thinks it's nerves trapped by scar tissue which may take months to right themselves. Keep on with the morphine, as 'the usual painkillers aren't effective with this kind of nerve-pain'. Can't face the Epiphany evening Eucharist. Too many kind enquiries expecting a more cheerful response than I can offer.

18th January

A bit stuck. It feels at times like going backwards. In such circumstances we cope better when we can divide up the time ahead into recognisable 'hoops' to jump through: (i) the pre-operation days of anxious anticipation; (ii) the operation and post op. trauma; (iii) the 32 sessions of radiotherapy; (iv) the time when the radiation is still powerfully active; (v) the weeks of the slow recovery of energy and the lessening of pain and discomfort; (vi) the achievement of new teeth. Mentally, you tick off the likely time each phase may take, but that 'likely' varies widely, and I seem trapped in stage (v). Not a case of 'been there; done that' which only works for (i) to (iii), but varies widely for each individual when it comes to (iv) to (vi). You just live in hope and think up ways of satisfying those who ask how you are which won't sound too negative.

Reading Kazuo Ishiguro's brilliant novel, *Never Let Me Go*, about a future in which children are cloned and bred solely to donate their organs to the seriously ill, and therefore doomed to die young. Which raises important questions about the direction experimentation with the human genome may take and what we mean by a human being.

19th January

To the clinic to see I.D. who feels I'm doing well, and says in the gentlest way that I must be more modest in my expectations. 'You've had a terrible disease, and terrible things have been done to you, both by me and in Southampton. It takes a year to recover from an aneurysm and this is just as devastating – in fact more invasive. You won't begin to feel yourself again for at least a year – and then you'll be a year older.' Point taken. He doesn't reckon to start on new teeth for at least six months. May have to do a bit of 'tidying up' first. Sounds ominous.

21st January

A beautiful, windless, sunny winter's day. To Roche Court sculpture park for a slow walk round. Henry Moore tapestries on show in the gallery. Wonderful light and shadows. First snowdrops just starting to open, an unlikely peacock butterfly, the distant cry of a buzzard, the smell of woodsmoke. The holy in the ordinary.

28th January

January has been lightened by three captivating books: A. N. Wilson's witty *tour de force* on life in the first half of the twentieth century, *After the Victorians*; and two novels, Jane Gardam's *Old Filth* and Jennifer Johnston's *Grace and Truth*, the first a funny, perceptive, moving picture of old age; the second a gripping and humane study of an outwardly failed life which explores the nature of grace and truth and the power of forgiveness.

29th January

I must begin to bring to an end this seven-month saga, adding a brief monthly summary and then some final thoughts when I can look back and see it in perspective, the pain behind me and the energy increased. I want to end on a high note and not a low one. What I most need now is patience, for my energy is still low, and the pain in the new jaw – ranging from a dull ache to something only morphine will hit – is persistent and unpredictable. I guess it still thinks it's a leg, but the metamorphosis will come. Each day has a certain sameness. Responding to enquiries gets harder. People expect a faster rate of improvement, but then so did I. January is a wearisome month at the best of times, and frustration a poor sort of tonic.

31st January: Reflecting on pain

'Pain in the mouth' writes Beryl Bainbridge, 'could be guaranteed to swamp every noble feeling known to man.'[114] Half an hour ago I was in pain: now I'm not. Morphine has intervened. Mind and body and the different sensory systems form an integrated whole, and the central nervous system receives constant reports of everything our ears, eyes, nose, mouth and body are experiencing. Pain is carried by electrical nerve impulses which travel along nerve fibres to the brain and signal to us that 'pain has occurred'. These may follow two pathways: the first, with fast conduction, is felt as a sharp sensation, like a pin-prick; the second as a slower, duller sensation, like a pinch. What my morphine has just done is not to interfere with the transmission of the pain impulses to the brain, but to alter the state of mind so that such impulses cause little distress. Anything to do with the brain is still a great mystery, and I shall come back to it in a final reflection on illness, simply thinking a little now on what exactly is going on in someone who feels pain. How cross we feel when it's suggested that an illness (M.E. is a good example) or pain is '*all* in the mind', where the implication seems to be that all of it is contained there and all of it, if not imaginary, is at least controllable. But if I *am* mind in this embodied spirit, this ensouled body, then the mystery of health and sickness and pain is far more profound and complex than that. And the vulnerability, the pain and the devastation we humans feel – as opposed to animals – in grief (say) is not a sign of weakness but of maturity and strength.

I've been helped to understand pain by a helpful book by Patrick Wall,[115] and from the insights of Dame Cicely Saunders in developing the hospice movement with its expertise in palliative care. Pain comes in all shapes and sizes and is as distinctive to the individual as is illness or faith or fingerprints. It is always personal, subjective, private. It needs to be understood as what Cicely Saunders calls 'total pain': physical, emotional, social and spiritual. It's experienced as a complete package, and depending on its context and severity brings with it feelings of fear and anxiety (generated by a sense of the unknown), unfairness and the need to protest, and the search for meaning: the question 'why?' as well as the question 'how do I cope with this?' Interestingly, Aristotle defined pain first and foremost as an emotion, and we use different kinds of words with which to describe it: *physical* words such as throbbing and crushing; *emotive* words such as frightening; words full of *meaning* such as cruel. (In a cancer research supplement in the *Guardian* people who had been affected by various forms of cancer were asked which were the most difficult aspects with which to deal. The figures were: practical effects 13%; physical effects 41%; emotional effects 45%. That's about right. To the question: have you experienced any difficulties in your relationship with husband, wife or partner as a result of your cancer diagnosis, 26% replied 'yes', a surprising 25% had actually broken up, and a further 12% had seriously considered it.)[116]

Pain focuses and monopolises our attention as few other states do and dominates our thinking. If we can relax in the face of it, know the cause of it and have an expectation of a successful outcome, these can all lessen the amount of pain we experience. Thus the extent of post-operative pain may be strongly affected by how much knowledge we are given beforehand of what is to be done to us, how much pain will be likely, where it will be, and how it will be controlled. Our pain thresholds differ greatly. While there is no basis for the common belief that men and women have different pain thresholds, individuals certainly do. Extroverts have a higher pain threshold than introverts, and anxiety is the strongest factor in determining how much pain we feel. Above all, pain can bring a sense of separation and a sense of unravelment, and it helps if it can be shared by those who, while unable to feel exactly what we're going through, are nevertheless prepared to listen so that we know that we aren't alone. Cicely Saunders once asked a patient what he chiefly looked for in those who were caring for him. He replied: 'For someone to look as if they are trying to understand me.' He didn't expect the impossible, just for an effort to empathise with how he felt and what he was going through. One of the things you most need in your doctors is not just that they will always explain, but that they will always listen.

February
proved a bleak month: biting winds, sub-zero temperatures, grey skies. Even the snowdrops were struggling. My mood matched it. The pain in the jaw increased, not so fiercely but for longer periods, as did the swelling and discomfort in the roof of the mouth, resisting the challenge of a second deep root canal and two spells of antibiotics. Became reluctant to talk much and hence to welcome friends, and even more reluctant to return to morphine, the only effective pain-killer. I.D. put me on Tegretol (given for epilepsy and tri-geminal neuralgia) which, in this litigious age, feels the need to list 75 possible side-effects, everything from deep-vein thrombosis to severe liver failure, via hallucinations, aggression and swelling of the breasts of both men and women. It ends, confortingly: 'Do not be alarmed by this. Most people take (the tablets) without any problems.' Just a certain wariness ... well deserved, as it turns out.

I.D. is puzzled by the pain, and at the end of the month

arranges a new CT scan. So we move into March somewhat anxiously.

March

Weather-wise, March was equally cold and bleak. Only on the 28th did it become a little warmer and the daffodils burst into flower. The scan, thank God, proved clear. A new X-ray showed some infection creeping up behind the two suspect teeth, failing to drain as the lymph nodes had either been removed or were only doing their job agonisingly slowly. So the teeth (on which I'd just spent a bomb on root canal treatment) were extracted, which in the still-traumatised mouth, with the radiation still lurking around, led to increased, prolonged pain. Referred to the pain clinic at the hospice, where Dr L. recommends a reluctant return to regular morphine. Delight comes as the month draws to a close, with the birth to M. and J. a few hours after Mothering Sunday of a son, Saul Benjamin. Who cares about some pain when you have a new grandchild?

Sarah and Chris Thorpe, so imaginative in their support during these months, send me John V. Taylor's appropriate poem, 'Lent':

> Jogging blind through winter's leaflessness
> we must last out this marathon of cold,
> though grime gathers under the grey duress
> and faith is grown old.
>
> Give back our springtime so the first petals' pink
> falls like alleluias through the melting air,
> deep in the loose loam let the gnarled roots drink
> and clenched ferns open to the sun in prayer.[117]

April

April proved 'the cruellest month'. It may have been the increase of morphine or (more likely) the larger doses of Tegretol that had been prescribed to counter the growing pain, but on the 13th, Maundy Thursday evening, as I got into bed, I lost control of my mind. Went completely dotty. I began talking not just jumbled-up words, but nonsense words, gobbledegook. I knew I was doing so but could do nothing to stop it. We always time these crises so well: the beginning of a long weekend with my doctor off-duty. The second stage was to start visualising individuals with acute vividness – every mole and wrinkle. None of them spoke: they simply arrived at the end of our bed, their eyes growing larger and more accusing. Over the next five days (all through Easter) the numbers grew, night and day; sometimes the small bedroom was crammed with up to 20 of them, all staring me down, and I felt too ill to get up. The plain wallpaper was transformed, the room decorated in a variety of exotic fashions, with a preference for pink French empire style with carved cornices, and I would be looking down at it from different angles of the ceiling.

There was, I discovered, one simple way of banishing these visitors: by holding their gaze and blinking hard. But it only worked for the current ones, and immediately others would appear. I grew fairly weak, and at times – such as when I found I was facing myself kneeling on the end of the bed in my dressing-gown and staring myself down – quite frightened too. All kinds of insects and messages appeared on the walls, as they had in hospital, although this was worse. Some messages were from people I had known. One persistent one appeared line by line in red ink, each line disappearing as a new line was written. There was nothing dream-like about the experience: I was wide awake throughout. At times I found papers in my hand, which dissolved as I began to read them, and on one occasion there was a large saucepan down the bed, which crumbled to dust. There were voices, and music, and in the small hours one of the innocent boys next door was penetrating the connecting wall by singing Second World War songs in a powerful bass voice. The duty doctor came and took me off all medication (including painkillers), and it was a relief to see G., our GP, back on Tuesday, who re-prescribed.

May: Final reflection on illness and healing

It may be a cliché that the most valuable lessons we have to learn come from our times of suffering, rather than from times of contentment, but it's profoundly true. Only an illusory religion offers a false hope of divine protection for those who belong to the right club. Many Christians discover in the face of grave illness or sudden grief that for a while their faith in God may make it harder, rather than easier, to come to terms with the experience; but in time a deep trust which is based on the conviction that there is a power of love sufficient for all our needs can give us a ground to which to hold firm. 'You must change your life,' wrote Rilke, and while you don't have to get cancer in order to look at life with new eyes, it certainly takes its place alongside leaving home, falling in love, or putting your faith in the Christlike God.

I've reflected on the isolating effect of illness, of how in some senses hospitals are unsuitable places in which to be ill. We underestimate the likely effect of stress and anxiety which lurks in these great impersonal buildings inevitably touched with indifference – however high the standard of care. In some parts of the States medical students are sent into hospital to spend a few days as patients incognito to gain some notion of what it's like. (It tends to be forgotten that 'hospital' and 'hospitality' and 'hospice' have the same root: the relationship of a host and a guest in a hostel or hotel.) Only a combination of confidence-giving technological expertise and compassion will take the sting out of your own aloneness. Even as a musician must know the exact technique of playing on a violin or a clarinet, and not just any old one but this distinctive one, even so each patient needs studying for his or her own characteristics and singularity. And where that level of perception happens, you know it.

'How are you?' 'Well,' we reply, or 'Not too bad,' when (so far as we can tell) every part of us, physical and psychological, is functioning in harmonious relationship with every other part and with our environment. When that relationship breaks down I say I'm feeling ill. Of course there's a subtle distinction between 'illness' and 'disease'. *Illness* is something beyond mere discomfort, but defined in *my* terms; *disease* is an objective clinical condition, independent of my judgement. So I may feel ill, rotten, 'run down'; but only the doctor can diagnose my disease. Which commonly leads to doctors having to focus on bits and pieces – microbes, hormone deficiencies, tumours, lungs, heart, ulcers – while I may experience my illness as the disorder, disruption and apparent disintegration of my life. And doctors may talk of treatment without distinguishing between the treatment of a *patient* and the treatment of a *disease*. To treat a disease is to inhibit it and hopefully help the body to destroy or control it: to treat a patient is to observe, foster, nurture and listen to a life. Most of the stories of Jesus' healing are the latter: most advice in medical textbooks the former. For the treatment of a disease is not an end in itself, but part of a larger process – that of becoming whole. The physicist David Bohm has written of how in Latin the root of the word 'whole' means both 'to cure' and also 'to measure', and he relates it very interestingly to the Platonic notion that every being, every thing, has its *right inward measure*; that a tree or a flower has its own quality of wholeness that gives it particular properties; that each human being has a right inward measure, when everything is balanced and physiologically homeostatic.[118] Medicine is the art of restoring that individual right inward measure when it has been forced off balance. Interestingly, in 1997 the World Health Organisation proposed that 'health' should be redefined as 'a dynamic state of complete physical, mental, *spiritual* and social well-being, not merely the absense of disease or infirmity'.

Yes, 'spiritual'. I am diminished if I have failed to explore, or have been prevented from exploring, the God-dimension in my life, diminished and consequently less whole as a human being. Health is a dynamic energy flow that changes over a lifetime. All our notions of health must be understood as such, as movement towards a goal: set in the context of the ultimate wholeness for which we were intended by a loving God. In the New Testament the Greek words for 'healing', 'health', 'wholeness' and 'salvation' are the same word, and the English words are interchangeable. Yet there are two quite different Greek words for 'healing' and 'curing'. The word for curing is used, for example, when Jesus cures the blind man by restoring his sight and tells his disciples: 'He was born blind that God's power might be displayed in curing him.' An example of the word for healing is when Paul prays that 'the sharp pain in his body might be removed' and gets the answer 'no'; he is firmly told that God's grace is all the healing he needs. In fact people with diseases at present incurable far outnumber those with curable ones, and if for us a full 'cure' physically or mentally is the overriding goal, then we shall regard our frequent inability to be so cured as failure – with dispiriting results. Yet people don't have to get out of their wheelchairs or terminal beds to show the presence of God's healing power in their lives. In such chronic or incurable illness the doctor's or the counsellor's healing role is first and foremost to reassure and restore the patient's integrity and worth.[119]

All this takes for granted the holistic approach to medicine, the modern understanding of this human wholeness to which the WHO definition refers. Body and mind can't be divided: indeed they are two ways of speaking of the same thing. This is particularly true of major breakdowns such as heart disease or cancer, which aren't infectious, yet (while it's true that a tiny minority of children contract cancer) it's how we live over a lifetime – how we think and feel – that can have a huge effect on such illnesses. Socrates came back from military service and reported to his fellow-countrymen 'that in one respect the barbarian Thracians were in advance of Greek civilisation. They knew that the body could not be cured without the mind.' In fact Aristotle had regarded body and mind as essentially inseparable, but in the seventeenth century Descartes argued powerfully and disastrously that mind and body are separate entities, united physically by the pineal gland. That paved the way for a damaging dualism that dealt a blow to the psychosomatic understanding of illness from which we are only just recovering. For years Freud tried to harmonise his view of mental illness with a purely mechanical model of disease, but discovered he was wrong. As the Bible writers knew. Bodies, considered physiologically and anatomically, need to have something added, and that something is an enlivening, activating breath or spirit in order that they may live. So, in the Genesis myth of creation God breathes into Adam the breath of life, in Hebrew *nephesh* (which can mean interchangeably 'breath' or 'life', 'soul' or 'mind'), and 'man became a living soul'. The Greek view was that man is an imprisoned spirit, the soul like a bird trapped in a cage; the very different Old Testament view is that each of us is an animated presence, a psychosomatic unity to whom God speaks and who can respond. In the New Testament the Greek words for body, flesh, spirit and mind (*soma*, *sarx*, *psyche* and *nous*) don't refer to distinctive bits of me, but always to the person that I am when viewed from a particular angle. Ultimately mysterious and indefinable, but one whose essence is in *being*, not having; and always with some mystery remaining.

Medical science is inevitably only concerned with what *is*, not what *ought* to be. Yet shouldn't we ask, not simply 'What are we?' but 'What might we be? If I believe that I am this embodied spirit created by (and called to respond to) God, then what *might* I be?' In an ideal NHS it would be good if every doctor and nurse in training would reflect on the mystery of the human being with both the learning of the scientist and the observation and sympathy of the novelist or the poet. The former tells me the mind-boggling facts about my body's 50 trillion unique cells, and how they may be sabotaged by cancer: the latter approaches the human mystery from a different angle. They know that things are simple or complex according to how much attention is paid to them. They know there is a kind of holiness about the body. They will not be surprised to read of the most unexpected developments with the increasingly detailed knowledge we now have of the nervous and hormonal systems and interactions within the cortex of the brain. Medical scientists, particularly in the great research hospitals of America, are searching for mechanisms that are much more complex than any simple dichotomy between mind and body. Time and again they point to the intimate connection between the nervous and the immune systems. Experiments are seeking to show that what a patient thinks and feels can strongly affect recovery, to discover what are the factors that impact on the brain, which then send signals that change the immune system. Some have shown, for example, that the suppression of grief and anger is associated with breast cancer in women, or congestive heart failure. They are clear that the brain which supplies all our intangible thoughts and feelings can cause a cascade of emotions in the body, and that it regulates the heart, the gastrointestinal system, the lungs, and probably the immune system. Neuroscientist David Felten of the University of Rochester School of Medicine, for example, has traced the nerve fibres that run like wires between the nervous system and the immune system. Every time we have a thought or feeling hormones are released that send a message to the immune system, and neurotransmitters are continuously talking to target cells throughout the body:

> We have this great [immune] defence system, which has a wonderful memory, and can generate responses to past [illnesses] that have come again. And we also have the brain with its wonderful memory of past experiences. We had thought these two great memory systems were independent. But now it turns out they're not – they talk to each other [all the time].[120]

It has been shown that one factor contributing to a diminished immune response is whether we feel isolated and lonely and whether or not we feel in control of a situation.

And of course, a change in the immune system makes a difference in the patient's disease. Felten writes of how

> One study at UCLA used actors who were told to think about a scenario, and generate in their own minds the feeling that came with it. While they did this, the hormones in their blood was tested, and you could see changes in some hormones and indications of subtle changes in their immune system, depending on what they were feeling.

Once the actor got out of the negative or positive state and was sitting quietly for half an hour, the immune system returned to normal. But I find the most fascinating research in this area that of Candace Pert, former Chief of the Brain Biochemistry Section of the American National Institute of Mental Health. She found that molecules called neuropeptides provide the crucial connection between mind and body. They are strung together like a string of pearls and act as messengers, travelling through every part of the body. They link with specific receptor molecules (which are like millions of satellite dishes all over each of our cells), as if guided by antennae tuned to the brain. And because their activity fluctuates with our state of mind, Pert calls these peptides the 'biochemical units of emotion': in other words, they translate our invisible emotions into visible bodily effects. It would have been unthinkable, 20 years ago, to claim that the cells of the immune system are constantly filtering through the brain and can actually lodge there. But Pert believes that the mind resides in the whole body, not just in the brain. She writes that 'the more we know of neuropeptides, the harder it is to think in traditional terms of mind and body. It makes more sense to speak of a single integrated unity, a body-mind.' That affirms what has formed the basis of Judaeo-Christian understanding of the human. Pert believes passionately that our moods and attitudes physically affect our organs and our tissues, and she even speaks of 'a form of energy that appears to leave the body when the body dies' to which she grudgingly gives the word 'spirit': 'We scientists', she says, 'are going to have to bring in ... the realm of spirit and soul that Descartes kicked out.' Asked where this trail leads us with regard to emotions and health, she replies:

> It leads us to think that the chemicals that are running our body and our brain are the same chemicals that are involved in emotion. And that says to me that we'd better seriously entertain theories about the role of emotions and emotional suppression in disease, and that we'd better pay more attention to emotions with regard to health.

Here, as elsewhere, there must be a new readiness to communicate between the professions; between the arts and the sciences; between doctors and theologians, professional and lay-person. That doesn't come naturally; in David Felten's phrase: 'We'd rather use each other's toothbrushes.' We use one kind of abstract language to describe the mind and another kind of material language to describe the body, languages that fail to connect, and this stops us seeing that these two kinds of phenomena are simply two manifestations of one process, and that mind, body and spirit are one and the same. For many scientists, we are no more than staggeringly complex electrochemical machines. Because there is no 'ghost in the machine', no clinically observable soul or spirit that exists independently of the body, there can be no self that will survive the body's disintegration. Our bodies, minds and consciousness, they say, evolved over hundreds of millions of years from primitive organisms, on a planet that formed from a gassy nebula about 4.5 million years ago. And in reply to the question *Why are we here?* they will say that we are here to make copies of our genes and thereby ensure the continuance of our species. Some forecast the day when we shall be able to explain artistic creativity as well as religious belief in terms of purely physical activity in the brain.

And yet it is only in us that the universe becomes conscious of itself: we alone can wonder at it and explore its secrets and be awed by its mystery. Each one of us is frail and vulnerable; too often we are to be discovered sitting in the doctor's waiting room, or lying in a hospital bed or on a psychiatrist's couch, crying out for healing. Crying out to be seen, not chiefly as a set of interesting symptoms or a machine requiring repair, but as a person, with all that word implies. Four hundred years ago John Donne wrote this in his *Devotions*:

> We study Health, and we deliberate upon our meats, and drink, and air, and exercises, and we hew, and we polish every stone that goes to that building; and so our health is a long and regular work; But in a minute a Canon batters all, overthrows all, demolishes all; a Sickness unprevented for all our diligence, unsuspected for all our curiosity; nay, undeserved, if we consider only disorder, summons us, seizes us, possesses us, destroys us in an instant.

Twice in my life this has happened to me. I have been knocked flat, trapped by illness and wonderfully diminished. But that reality conjures up the dominant story in the Christian life, its great redeeming truth: that of the wounded healer (Eliot's 'wounded surgeon'); the one made incarnate and laid low, sharing our vulnerability, our encounter with mystery, our Job-like search for answers; the one who encounters our mystery and himself enters into our troubled questions. And in his light, we are helped to see light; and to endure.

POSTSCRIPT: ASCENSIONTIDE

A few months ago I had thought that (as in all the best fairy-tales) there would be a happy ending. But life is not like that. There are no Q.E.D.s. Instead we live in hope, that orientation of the spirit which serves as a guard against depression and is a persuasive companion of faith and love; hope that in the end 'all shall be well, and all manner of thing shall be well'. We live in a world in which, in that tiresome phrase, 'bad things happen to good people'. ('Define "good".') One in which the rain falls on the just and the unjust; and prayers are answered in unexpected ways.

And there *is* no conventional 'happy ending' for me. The biopsy taken a fortnight ago has come back positive. To everyone's surprise the cancer has returned, and the options now are limited. This doesn't change anything I have written, though I shall want to add some final reflections over the next week or two. I have had the welcome if unwanted privilege of taking a fresh look at my life: of learning more about its meaning, about myself and about those I love. Following the discipline of Lent, the continuing endurance of Passiontide and the anguish of the cross, I mustn't overlook all the signs of Easter. Fully aware that on the risen body of Jesus the scars from the scourging, the nail-marks and the piercing remain and are recognised as the test and proof of his humanity.

The epistle set for Ascension Day speaks to me. Paul's Letter to the Ephesians 1:18-19a:

> I pray that your inward eyes may be enlightened, so that you may know what is the hope to which (God) calls you, how rich and glorious is the share he offers you among his people in their inheritance, and how vast are the resources of his power open to us who have faith.

243

And that is backed up by those familiar words from the Benedictus, in which Zechariah foretells how his son John will prepare the way for Jesus, of how in him

> In the *tender compassion* of our God,
>> the *dawn* from on high *shall break upon us,*
>> *To shine on those who dwell in darkness and the shadow of death,*
>> and to guide our feet into the way of *peace.*[1]

*

I go into what now look like my final weeks or months knowing that I don't go alone, but supported by family and friends, and undergirding us the three religious communities of West Malling, Tymawr and Burford. In a sense, this book is offered to all who are holding A. and me in their thoughts and prayers: those three Benedictine communities; prayer groups in my former parishes of Norton, Letchworth and Great St Mary's, Cambridge; many at Westminster Abbey; friends from every phase of my life; my attentive, thoughtful, lovable family; Gerry Hughes, with his generous foreword; the clergy and people of Salisbury Cathedral. You know who you are: what you can only guess at is my profound gratitude. Nor do I forget my two latest grandchildren, Ella and Saul. They won't have any memory of their grandfather, but should be in no doubt of the delight their birth has brought me. (And how good it was, Saul, later in July to have just enough energy left to enable me to baptise you.) A delight that has been so amply fulfilled in my other grand-children, Adam and Anna, both so gifted and so sensitive to my condition in this past year.

I am grateful, too, to all the members of the medical team who have looked after me with such skill, even though their efforts were to be frustrated in the end; to St Christopher's Hospice (of which I am Honorary Vice-President and which I served for sixteen years as a Trustee), Barbara Monroe (its Chief Executive) and Dr Victor Pace, for taking me in for a week in May to monitor and advise on pain control; to Graham, my dedicated GP, and Sheila, gentlest of practice nurses during long weeks of daily dressing; to the dedicated team of nurses at Salisbury Hospice (S. H.), working alongside Christine its Medical Director, Sharon my hospice doctor, and Annie, Community Palliative Care Sister. And not least, to Brendan Walsh, editorial director, and the staff at Darton, Longman and Todd, for a great act of affirmation in commissioning this book sight unseen.

Each of us learns – or fails to learn – from illness in our own way. What I have learned is that, while God may often seem remote and your faith less resistant than you would wish, yet that Kingdom-melody which has been fashioned in me over a lifetime has survived and has proved a strength. I have sought to keep faith with the Psalmist: *My heart is firmly fixed, O God, my heart is fixed; I will sing, and make melody.*[2] The melody that endures. I have learned that in a crisis God's grace works through the kindness and thoughtfulness of the countless people whose lives we have touched, hopefully (and often unawares) for the good. I have learned a little more of what the cost of marriage may be for my wife and loved ones, as together we explore the demands of 'in sickness and in health'. I have grown in admiration for the skill and dedication of the best in the medical profession. I have learned how scary it can be when drugs stifle your reason and leave you confused and drowning in a world adrift somewhere between logic and nonsense.

These ten months have been unlike any others I have known. Many people have helped redeem them, and not least the discipline (and therapy) of writing, the pleasure of reading, and the observing of the changing seasons. Which is to say: the communication of what it feels like to be part and parcel of this messy, unpredictable, often distressing but always beautiful world. 'May we (learn to) see', writes Vikram Seth at the very end of *Two Lives*, 'that we could have been born as each other.' Which takes me back to where I started in the Introduction: of how, out of the sharing of our vulnerability, empathy grows. However mixed our motives in writing (or reading) books, in the end they are about our desire to share (and learn more about) what it means to be human and what matters to us most, our desire to 'speak what we feel, not what we ought to say'[3]. For those who write such books, and nervously launch them into a critical world, they aim to be, in short, a small – and sometimes quite risky – act of love.

I don't intend to spin things out. What lies ahead (which turned out to include the inability to eat and the insertion of a stomach feeding tube; damage to the cornea of my good 'reading eye' – very demoralising; and the rapid growth of cancerous nodules in the neck, demanding daily dressings) contains times best kept private, and I don't want to unbalance what I have written. For the truth of what has happened in this past year as I've tried to describe it is unaltered by the outcome. Instead I simply want to add a tiny handful of vignettes which for different reasons have proved important and life-enhancing. For that's what they're all about, these last days: not the *amount* of time left to me but its *quality*, the living of this earthly life as fully as possible to the end. When Philip Toynbee was dying, he remembered how a young priest had told him that he had been ordained because 'I wanted a job where I couldn't feel the bottom'. And Toynbee comments that dying will be that sort of job too.

*

Judy R. takes us to spend the morning with Vikram S. in George Herbert's rectory in Bemerton. I long to stand in Herbert's house and garden one more time. V. and I take chairs and sit by the river Nadder. We drink green tea and talk about Herbert, but more widely about poetry and redressing the balance and what in life proves of lasting value; about the nature of goodness and the power of empathy. I ask him to read for me Herbert's astonishing small poem which so powerfully conveys the nature of God's gracious love, *Love bade me welcome*. He has no need to read it: he recites it by heart. Eighteen lines which change for ever any false concept of a dominant, authoritarian God into that of one who serves and invites us to let him wait on us. ('You must sit down', says Love, 'and taste my meat.' / So I did sit and eat.) A poem that did more than anything else to convert Simone Weil to the Christian faith. Talking to V. about my book, and my realisation that I may well not live to see it published in five months' time, he reminds me that Herbert, like Gerard Manley Hopkins, died without seeing his poems in print: indeed, without knowing whether or not they would ever be published.

We tour the house, each room now having a different theme: the music room with its piano, scores and books on the composers; the Indian room, with its books on the Hindu scriptures; George Herbert's bedroom, filled with poetry. I sit alone for a few minutes in the room in which he died after three short years of parish ministry to the people of Bemerton and Fugglestone, during which he laid down the pattern for the model Anglican priest. V. gives us a jar of medlar jelly, and a sprig of medlar from a tree in whose shade we sat. Its white flower is like that of a small magnolia. It used to be planted, along with quince, mulberry and walnut, at the four corners of herb gardens and orchards.

Searching Herbert's complete works for *Love* (3), the book fell open at a poem I had never consciously read entitled *Death*. The reference to 'Half that we have' in the last verse is the half of life not spent in sleep, and Herbert is saying that we might as well die, as sleep. It matters not whether we find our rest in the *down* of pillows, or the *dust* of the grave.

Death, thou wast once an uncouth hideous thing,
    Nothing but bones,
   The sad effect of sadder groans:
Thy mouth was open, but thou couldst not sing.

For we consider'd thee as at some six
    Or ten years hence,

After the loss of life and sense,
Flesh being turn'd to dust, and bones to sticks.

We lookt on this side of thee, shooting short
      Where we did find
    The shells of fledge* souls left behind
Dry dust, which sheds no tears, but may extort.

But since our Saviour's death did put some blood
      Into thy face,
    Thou art grown fair and full of grace,
Much in request, much sought for, as a good.

For we do now behold thee gay and glad,
      As at dooms-day,
    When souls shall wear their new array,
And all thy bones with beauty shall be clad.

Therefore we can go die as sleep, and trust
      Half that we have
    Unto an honest faithful grave;
Making our pillows either down, or dust.

    *fledge: fully plumed and able to fly

*****

When I stood before my bishop at my ordination fifty years ago the Ordination Charge was read. It contained these words: 'You are to teach and encourage by word and example ... and you are *to prepare the dying for their death* ... ' Donald Nicholl, in his *The Testing of Hearts*, where he keeps a diary of his final weeks, writes of what it means to go on 'witnessing to the end'. Of what is he to witness? Not to his ability to 'die a good death', but to witness to the grace of God, his continuing Presence. 'Now is the time for me to *validate* everything that I have claimed as true either by my sermons and addresses, or my writings and actions.'[4] The hardest thing for me at present is to accept an unpleasant open wound in the throat, which will continue to grow and which needs a daily dressing by the nurse; and it possesses the worst scent in the world, the smell of cancer. That's the kind of unpredictable development which comes to dominate the day. I find myself saying more and more: 'I can do all things through Christ who strengthens me.'

Prayers become simplified. Each morning I say a slightly truncated daily office from *Celebrating Common Prayer*, using one psalm and one New Testament lesson. In the evening I simply make a final act of committal of myself and my loved ones and the day, something like this:

> Abba – Father – Creator – Sustainer: source and fulfilment of all that I am. You hold me in your presence and enfold me in your love: hold me in and through my dying and raise me to new life.
>
> Thank you for this day, for love given and received …
>
> For beauty and for goodness …
>
> I pray for those I love, especially … that we may have courage and endurance in what lies ahead.
>
> I give myself into your hands this night: may I be free from anxiety and pain and bad dreams.
>
> Father, I will lay me down in peace, for it is you, Lord, only who makes me dwell in safety. Into your hands I commend my spirit, for you have redeemed me, O Lord God of truth.

*

Graham, our GP, back from New Zealand, visits. As he leaves I say how grateful we are that we are being cared for by such a good team. 'And don't forget,' he replies, 'that you're the team leader.'

A truth made only too apparent when Sarah, A. and I go to Southampton a few days later for the result of the latest scan. It is not good. It shows two cancerous growths, the size of 10-penny pieces, under the chin, almost certainly stemming from the primary cancer, which has eluded the radiotherapy. I feel so sorry for Ian, whose remarkable surgery has come to nothing. The cancer will continue to grow, though at what rate is anyone's guess. The options are very limited. The radiotherapy was so fierce that it can't be repeated; surgery would not work, as a wound would not heal; I have said 'no' to aggressive chemotherapy. That leaves the possibility of a milder form of the latter: a weekly injection and pills after 24 hours to counteract the poison. Side-effects are likely to be tiredness, nausea, and 'gritty' eyes. It works in one out of four cases, and might lead to a few more months of life. We have a few days to think it over, but I know already what we'll opt for. Quality, not quantity of days.

Even though I knew this would be the outcome, there is still a sense of shock in hearing it spelled out so finally, and part of me wants to weep and feels nothing but fear and dismay. And with A., from time to time, I am wracked by sobs which indicate just what lies under the attempt at a brave face. In the psalmist's words:

> My spirit faints within me; my heart within me is desolate.
>
> I remember the time past...I consider the works of your hands ...
>
> O Lord, make haste to answer me; my spirit fails me; hide not your face from me
>
> > lest I be like those who go down to the Pit.[5]

When he was dying of a rapid cancer my friend and colleague Giles Ecclestone spoke of his attempt to view his death as 'a gift'. That's hard; some will think even a bit perverse. And yet he was entirely right. Our lives are sheer gift, as is the creation, and that our little lives are 'rounded with a sleep' as they transmute from one phase to the next (whatever that may be) is as natural as being born. We each choose to die in our own way, though for some it will be harder than for others, but if we can see it as 'gift', then it will be so insofar as we face it in such a way as to draw good out of it; trying (however reluctantly, however painfully) to deliberately unseal our clenched fists and let go of what we have been given with open hands. To die with gratitude for all that has been, without resentment for what you are going through, and with openness towards the future, is the greatest gift we can leave those who love us and who are left behind.

I can't think of a better ending than some words from the first book written by a lifelong friend, John Austin Baker, for they say it all.

> I rest on God, who will assuredly not allow me to find the meaning of life in his love and forgiveness, to be wholly dependent on him for the gift of myself, and then destroy that meaning, revoke that gift. He who holds me in existence now can and will hold me in it still, through and beyond the dissolution of my mortal frame. For this is the essence of love, to affirm the right of the beloved to exist. And what God affirms, nothing and no-one can contradict.[6]

*****

In these past weeks I have been pondering on the ordered rhythm of the seasons. The swifts are back, threading the air; the woods are dappled with wild blossom and the gardens full of the scent of lilac; the thrush claims his territory, early and late; the hedgerows are hung with May. Each witnesses to change, to the annual pattern of death and new life. Each summons us to a sense of wonder at nature's *cantus firmus*. A melody that is both hopeful and enduring.

NOTES

1. W. B. Yeats, 'The Municipal Gallery Revisited VII', *The Collected Poems* (Everyman, J. M. Dent, 1992).
2. W. B. Yeats, 'A Prayer for Old Age', *The Collected Poems, op. cit.*
3. William Boyd, *The New Confessions* (Penguin, 1988).
4. John Donne, *Devotions* (1624), *Complete Poetry and Selected Prose* (Nonesuch Press, 1929).

Introduction
1. George Eliot, *Adam Bede* (Everyman, J. M. Dent, 1992).
2. *Guardian*, 12.09.01.
3. *Observer*, interview with Kate Kellaway, 16.09.01.

PART I: The *Cantus Firmus*
1. Patrick White, *Riders in the Chariot* (Penguin, 1964).
2. Dietrich Bonhoeffer, *Letters and Papers from Prison* (SCM Press, 1953).
3. William Byrd, Preface to *Gradualia* (1607).
4. David Bentley Hart, *The Beauty of the Infinite* (Eerdmans, 2004).
5. John Heath-Stubbs, 'Homage to J. S. Bach', *Selected Poems* (Carcanet, 1990).
6. Dietrich Bonhoeffer, *Letters and Papers from Prison, op. cit.*
7. R. S. Thomas, 'Suddenly', *Collected Poems 1945–1990* (Dent, 2000).
8. John Donne, 'Hymne to God my Father in my Sicknesse', *Divine Poems* (OUP, 1982).
9. Immanuel Kant, *Critique of Practical Reason*, Conclusion (1787).
10. John Donne, *Divine Poems*, XV.
11. Ron Ferguson and Mark Chater, *Mole Under the Fence: Conversations with Roland Walls* (St Andrew Press, 2006).
12. Gregory Dix, *The Shape of the Liturgy* (Dacre Press,1945).
13. George Steiner, *Errata: An Examined Life* (Weidenfield & Nicholson, 1997).
14. George Tyrrell, quoted in Nicholas Sagovsky, *On God's Side* (OUP, 1990).
15. Bernard Levin, article in *The Times*, 24.12.62. Reproduced in *I Should Say So* (Jonathan Cape, 1995).

PART II: The Time of Harvest
1. Rainer Maria Rilke, 'Duino Elegies VIII', *Selected Poetry* (Vintage International, 1989).

2. D. J. Enright, 'Memory', *Old Men and Comets* (OUP, 1993).
3. W. H. Auden, 'Lullaby', *Thank You, Fog* (Faber, 1974).
4. Bill Bryson, *A Short History of Nearly Everything*, Introduction (Black Swan, 2004).
5. Anthony Hecht, 'Peripateia', *Millions of Strange Shadows* (New York, Athenaeum 1977).
6. John Mortimer, *The Summer of a Dormouse* (Viking, 2000).
7. *As You Like It*, Act II, Scene vii.
8. Isaiah 46:3-4 in Jerusalem Bible.
9. Michel de Montaigne, 'Essay, Book 1, no. 19', *Collected Essays* (Penguin, 1958).
10. Marilynne Robinson, *Gilead* (Virago, 2005).
11. Philip Larkin, 'The Old Fools', *Collected Poems* (Faber, 1988).
12. Jamie McKendrick, 'Give or Take', *Ink Stone* (Faber, 2003).
13. Graham Swift, *The Light of Day* (Penguin, 2003).
14. Helen M. Luke, *Old Age* (New York, Parabola Books, 1987).
15. Alan Bennett, *The History Boys* (Faber, 2004).
16. Anton Chekhov, Olga in *Three Sisters*, Act IV (Methuen, 2000).
17. Anthony Hecht, essay on Charles Simic in *Melodies Unheard* (John Hopkins, 2003).
18. Lord Byron, *Letters & Journals*, 12 vols., ed. Leslie A. Marchand (John Murray, 1973–82).
19. T. S. Eliot, 'Little Gidding', *The Four Quartets*.
20. Raymond Carver, 'Late Fragment', from *All of Us* (Harvill Press, 1996).
21. Eric Abbott, *The Compassion of God and the Passion of Christ* (Geoffrey Bles, 1963).
22. *Hamlet*, Act V, Scene ii.
23. *King Lear*, Act V, Scene iii.
24. Ecclesiastes 12:5–8.
25. Edith Sitwell, 'Eurydice', *Collected Poems* (Macmillan, 1957).

PART III: The Questioning Country of Cancer

1. Christopher Fry, *A Yard of Sun* (OUP, 1970).
2. Alexander Pope, Epistle i, 1, 13.
3. *The Letters of Sydney Smith*, ed. Nowell C. Smith (OUP, 1981).
4. Hugh Dickinson, version of Psalm 119, privately circulated.
5. Rainer Maria Rilke, *Book of Hours: Love Poems to God*, I, 19, trans. Barrows & Macy (New York, Riverhead Books, 1996).
6. *Ibid.*, III, 1.
7. *Ibid.*, I, 1.
8. W. H. Auden, 'Musée des Beaux Arts', *Collected Shorter Poems* (Faber, 1950).
9. Letter from Hugh Dickinson to Michael Mayne, August 2005.
10. All quotations from Ian Mackenzie's script of 14.8.05, used with permission.
11. Daniel Barenboim and Edward Said, *Parallels and Paradoxes: Explorations in Music and Society* (Bloomsbury, 2003).

12. *Ibid.*, p. 44.
13. *Ibid.*, pp. 141, 165.
14. Philippians 1:21–24.
15. J. A. T. Robinson, sermon preached in Trinity College Chapel, Cambridge, 23.10.83.
16. Bill Moyers, *Healing and the Mind* (New York, Doubleday, 1993).
17. D. H. Lawrence, *Selected Letters*, Inroduction by Aldous Huxley (Penguin, 1950).
18. R. S. Thomas, 'Suddenly', *Collected Poems 1945–1990* (Dent, 2000).
19. Andrew Marvell, 'Upon Appleton House', *Complete Poems* (Viking, 1977).
20. Tom Lubbock, *Guardian*, 19.8.05.
21. *King Lear*, Act IV, Scene ii.
22. Thomas Hardy, 'De Profundis', *'Wessex' and 'Past & Present Poems'* (Macmillan, 1908).
23. Edwin Muir, *The Story and the Fable* (Hogarth Press, 1940).
24. Kathleen Jamie, *Findings* (Sort Of Books, Penguin, 2005).
25. Carol Ann Duffy, 'Prayer', *Selected Poems* (Penguin, 1994).
26. Alan Bennett, *The History Boys*, Act 2 (Faber, 2004).
27. Sally Purcell, 'Poem for Lent or Advent' (Anvil Press Poetry, 2002).
28. Don Paterson, 'Rhyme and Reason', *Guardian*, 6.11.04.
29. *London Review of Books*, 7.7.05.
30. John Burnside, 'Kith', *The Light Trap* (Cape Poetry, 2002).
31. Karen Armstrong, *The Battle for God: Fundamentalism in Judaism, Christianity and Islam* (HarperCollins, 2000).
32. George Steiner, *Errata: An Examined Life* (Weidenfield & Nicholson, 1997).
33. 1 John 1:1–2.
34. *Doctrine in the Church of England* (SPCK, 1922).
35. Romans 4:17.
36. T. F. Torrance, *Space, Time and Incarnation* (OUP, 1969).
37. Rowan Williams, 'Poetic and Religious Imagination', *Theology*, May 1977 (SPCK).
38. Dylan Thomas, *Collected Poems* (J. M. Dent, 1952).
39. William Blake, 'The Little Black Boy', *Songs of Innocence & Experience* (Chatto & Windus, 1938).
40. Richard Hoggart, *First and Last Things* (Aurum Press, 1999).
41. John 15:14–15.
42. Terry Eagleton, 'Living in a Material World', *Guardian*, 20.9.03.
43. Margaret Atwood, *Alias Grace* (Virago, 1997).
44. Aubrey's *Brief Lives*, ed. Oliver Lawson Dick (Peregrine, 1949).
45. D. H. Lawrence, 'There is nothing to see', *Complete Poems* (Penguin, 1993).
46. John McGahern, *Memoir* (Faber, 2005).
47. Mary Kenny, *The Literary Review*, Sept. 2005.
48. Cecil Torr, *Small Talk at Wreyland* (OUP, 1979).
49. Peter Kane Dufault, 'Evensong', *Looking in All Directions* (Worple Press, 2000).

50. Sylvia Townsend Warner, 30.xii.58, *Letters*, ed. William Maxwell (Chatto & Windus, 1982).

51. Michael McCrum, *The Man Jesus: Fact and Legend* (Janus, 1999).

52. John Donne, *Sermon to the Nativity*.

53. *Hamlet*, Act V, Scene ii.

54. Frederick Buechner, *The Faces of Jesus* (Stearn/Harper & Row, 1974).

55. William Law, *Fire From a Flint*, daily readings, ed. Robert Llewelyn & Edward Moss (DLT, 1986).

56. Ivan Turgenev, *Dream Tales and Prose Poems*, trans. Edward Garnett (Heinemann, 1897).

57. Quoted in E. L. Allen, *Freedom in God* (Hodder & Stoughton, 1950).

58. Alan Ecclestone, *Yes to God* (DLT, 1975).

59. Isaiah 7:13.

60. William Blake, *The Everlasting Gospel*, i, 13.

61. Owen Chadwick, *The Reformation* (Penguin, 1990).

62. Ronan Bennett, *Havoc, in the Third Year* (Review, 2005).

63. Quoted in Malcolm Barnes, *Augustus Hare, a Victorian Gentleman* (Allen & Unwin, 1984).

64. Will Hutton, 'Thank God for Rowan Williams', *Observer*, 8.12.02.

65. Alice Meynell, 'The Unknown God', *The Poems of Alice Meynell* (Burns, Oates & Washbourne, 1924).

66. Alan Ecclestone, *Gather the Fragments* (Sheffield, Cairns Publications, 1993).

67. John McPhee, *Basin and Range* (Farrar, Strauss & Giroux, 1980), quoted in Bill Bryson, *A Short History of Nearly Everything* (Black Swan, 2004), from which I have taken these scientific details.

68. Philip Larkin, 'Aubade', *Collected Poems* (Faber, 1988).

69. George Eliot, *Adam Bede* (Everyman, J. M. Dent, 1992).

70. *Letters of John Keats*, ed. Robert Giddings (OUP, 1970).

71. Milan Kundera, speech made at reception of Jerusalem Prize for Peace, 1985.

72. Jeanette Winterson, essay in *Reading for Pleasure*, ed. Antonia Fraser (Bloomsbury, 1992).

73. George Steiner, *Real Presences* (Faber, 1989).

74. Andrei Makine, *Le Testament Francais*, trans. Geoffrey Strachan (Hodder & Stoughton, 1997).

75. Seamus Heaney, *Finders Keepers: Atlas of Civilisation* (Faber, 2002).

76. Zbigniew Herbert, *Report from the Besieged City*, trans. John Carpenter & Bogdana Carpenter (OUP, 1985).

77. Seamus Heaney, 'Secular and Millennial Milosz', *Finders Keepers*, *op. cit.*

78. Donald Rayfield, *Stalin and His Hangmen* (Viking, 2004).

79. Wallace Stevens, 'The Noble Rider and the Sound of Words', lecture at Princeton University, 1941.

80. Vaclav Havel, 'Six Asides about Culture', *Living in Truth* (Faber, 1987).

81. Interview with Bill Moyers in *The Language of Life: A Festival of Poets* (Doubleday, 1995).

82. George Steiner, 'English Tomorrow', *After Babel* (OUP, 1975).

83. R. S. Thomas, 'Don't ask me', *Residues* (Bloodaxe, 2002).

84. See John Armstrong, *The Secret Power of Beauty* (Penguin, 2005).

85. P. T. Forsyth, *Religion in Recent Art* (London, 1905).

86. St Augustine, *Confessions* (London, 1961).

87. J. V. Taylor, *The Christlike God* (SCM Press, 1992).

88. Evelyn Underhill, *Mysticism* (Methuen, 1911).

89. Quotations from Peter Fuller, *Theoria: Art and the Absence of Grace* (Chatto & Windus, 1988).

90. Words quoted at an exhibition of her work at the St Ives Tate Gallery, 2004.

91. John Berger, *The White Bird* (London, 1985).

92. George Steiner, *Real Presences, op. cit.*

93. John Donne, 'Sermon at the Funeral of Sir William Cokayne' (1626).

94. *Anthony and Cleopatra*, Act V, Scene ii.

95. Jean-Pierre de Caussade, *The Flame of Divine Love*, ed. Robert Lewellyn (DLT, 1984).

96. Patrick Kavanagh, quoted in *Guardian* article by Robert Macfarlane, 30.7.05.

97. Don Paterson, *The Book of Shadows* (Picador, 2004).

98. U. A. Fanthorpe, 'BC/AD', *Standing To* (Peterloo, 1982).

99. Richard Crashaw, 'Hymn of the Nativity' from *Quem Vidistis Pastores* in *Complete Works*, ed. L. C. Martin (OUP, 1927).

100. Jürgen Moltmann, *Theology of Hope* (SCM Press, 1967).

101. See Chapter 2 of my book, *Learning to Dance*!

102. 2 Corinthians 4:18.

103. Dennis Potter, interview with Melvyn Bragg, Channel 4, April 1994.

104. John Stewart Collis, *Bound Upon a Course* (Sidgwick & Jackson, 1971).

105. Dietrich Bonhoeffer, *Letters and Papers from Prison* (SCM Press, 1953).

106. John McGahern, *Memoir, op. cit.*

107. Quoted in Edward Schillebeeckx, *Jesus, An Experiment in Christology* (Collins, 1979).

108. Sir Isaac Newton, quoted in L. T. More, *Isaac Newton* (1934).

109. Quoted in *The Faber Book of Science*, ed. John Carey (Faber, 1995).

110. Hosea 6:3-4.

111. St Augustine, Sermon 241.2.2, quoted in *The Heart at Rest* (DLT, 1986).

112. Jonathan Sacks, *To Heal a Fractured World* (Continuum, 2005).

113. Padraig J. Daly, 'Trinity', *The Other Sea* (Dublin, Dedalus Press, 2003).

114. Beryl Bainbridge, *Watson's Apology* (Penguin, 1992).

115. Patrick Wall, *Pain, the Science of Suffering* (Weidenfeld & Nicolson, 1999).

116. *Guardian*, 8.4.06.

117. John V. Taylor: 'Lent', *A Christmas Sequence & Other Poems* (Amate Press, 1989).

118. David Bohm, *Wholeness and the Implicate Order*, quoted in Bill Moyers, *Healing and the Mind, op. cit.*

119. I am greatly indebted to the writing of the great French Christian doctor, Pierre Tournier.

120. Bill Moyers, *Healing and the Mind*, *op. cit.*

Postscript: Ascensiontide

1. Luke 1:78–79.

2. Psalm 57:7.

3. *King Lear*, Act V, Scene iii.

4. Donald Nicholl, *The Testing of Hearts* (Darton, Longman and Todd, 1998).

5. Psalm 143: 4–7.

6. John Austin Baker, *The Foolishness of God* (Darton, Longman and Todd, 1970).

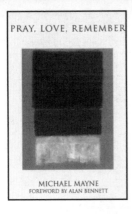
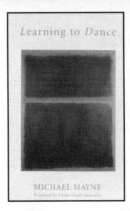
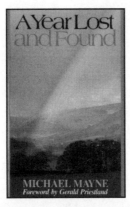